Leisure Opportunities for Individuals with Disabilities: Legal Issues

Susan J. Grosse
Donna Thompson
Editors

Sponsored by the
**Adapted Physical Activity Council of the
Association for Research, Administration,
Professionals Councils and Societies**

An association of the
**American Alliance for Health, Physical Education,
Recreation and Dance**

The American Alliance for Health, Physical Education, Recreation and Dance is an educational organization designed to support, encourage, and provide assistance to member groups and their personnel nationwide as they initiate, develop, and conduct programs in health, leisure, and movement-related activities. The Alliance seeks to:

- Encourage, guide, and support professional growth and development in health, leisure, and movement-related programs based on individual needs, interests, and capabilities.
- Communicate the importance of health, leisure, and movement-related activities as they contribute to human well-being.
- Encourage and facilitate research which will enrich health, leisure, and movement-related activities and to disseminate the findings to professionals and the public.
- Develop and evaluate standards and guidelines for personnel and programs in health, leisure, and movement-related activities.
- Coordinate and administer a planned program of professional, public, and government relations that will improve education in areas of health, leisure, and movement-related activities.
- Conduct other activities for the public benefit.

Contents

Foreword

Now, as never before, individuals (of all ages) with disabilities (of all kinds) are engaging in leisure activities. As a result, program providers are faced with unique challenges. Quality instruction in leisure activity skills is important. However, instruction is meaningless if a program is not accessible to anyone who wishes to participate, if program information is not available to all interested individuals, if activity inherent risks are not managed in an appropriate manner, if safety standards are not followed, or if industry regulations are not observed.

This publication explores legal issues serving as foundations for quality active leisure participation by individuals with disabilities. The Alliance initially provided instructional resources through the Unit on Programs for the Handicapped and its Information and Research Utilization Center by publishing the Practical Pointer monograph series. This book, developed through support of the Adapted Physical Activity Council, continues the tradition of that practical information. In addition to documenting implementation details of the Americans with Disabilities Act (ADA), playground and equipment standards and guidelines, and American Camping Association standards, specific information is presented on risk management, liability, negligence, and accessibility.

The authors have infused technical and theoretical information with practical application and examples. We are grateful to them for sharing their expertise and commitment. Written for professionals charged with program implementation, but equally valuable as a resource for administrators, this publication bears the mark of Julian U. Stein, originator of the Practical Pointer concept and long champion for individuals with disabilities and those who provide programs for them. Our sincere thanks to Dr. Stein and also to Dr. Raymond A. Ciszek, of the Alliance, who helped bring this project to its conclusion.

Users of this publication will also be interested in its companion volume, *Play and Recreation for Individuals with Disabilities: Practical Pointers*, another project of the Adapted Physical Activity Council, which focuses on teaching ideas for the many new opportunities now challenging individuals with disabilities.

SUSAN J. GROSSE
DONNA THOMPSON

About the Authors

Annie Clement, PhD, JD, is a professor at Cleveland State University, Cleveland, Ohio.

Tom Collier is camp director of Camp ASCCA (Alabama Special Camp for ChiLdren and Adults), Jackson Gap, Alabama.

Eric Dresser is program director of Camp ASCCA (Alabama Special Camp for Children and Adults), Jackson Gap, Alabama.

Ann E. Graziadei is assistant professor in physical education and recreation at Gallaudet University, Washington, DC.

Susan J. Grosse, formerly on staff at Gaenslen Orthopedic School in Milwaukee, Wisconsin, teaches physical education at the Milwaukee High School of the Arts.

Jill Hembree is a certified recreation therapist at Lakeshore Rehabilitation Complex, Birmingham, Alabama.

Susan F. McConnell teaches physical education for the Milwaukee Public Schools. She is a former Girl Scout camp director and presently serves the American Camping Association as a member of its Board of Visitors.

James V. Mastro, PhD, is a research fellow in the Minnesota Rehabilitation Research Training Program, Institute on Community Integration, University of Minnesota.

Barbara M. Moody is a physical education instructor, Andrew Johnson Elementary School, Kingsport, Tennessee.

David N. Reams, PhD, is adapted physical education supervisor for Dade County Public Schools, Florida.

Delores Richmond is principal of Andrew Johnson Elementary School, Kingsport, Tennessee.

Glen M. Roswal, PhD, is professor of health, physical education, and recreation at Jacksonville State University, Alabama.

Mark Singleton is marketing vice president of Nantahala Outdoor Center, Bryson City, North Carolina.

Julian U. Stein, PhD, formerly director of the Information and Research Utilization Center, Unit on Programs for the Handicapped, American Alliance for Health, Physical Education, Recreation and Dance, is retired professor of physical education, George Mdason University, residing in Oliver Springs, Tennessee.

Todd Teske is coordinator of special services for the Eau Claire Area School District, Eau Claire, Wisconsin.

Donna Thompson, PhD, is associate professor of health, physical education, and recreation, University of Northern Iowa, Cedar Falls.

Timothy P. Winter, PhD, is associate professor of physical education and health at Idaho State University, Pocatello.

James B. Wise is a certified recreation therapist and director of the Cooperative Wilderness Handicapped Outdoor Group (C.W. Hog) at Idaho State University, Pocatello.

Sue C. Wortham, PhD, is professor, Division of Education, University of Texas at San Antonio.

Section One

LEGAL CONCERNS

The Americans with Disabilities Act:
Implications for Recreation and Leisure

Julian U. Stein

The Americans with Disabilities Act (ADA) was signed into law by President George Bush on July 26, 1990, and put into effect on January 26, 1992. It "establishes a clear and comprehensive federal prohibition of discrimination against persons with disabilities in private sector employment and ensures equal access for persons with disabilities to public accommodations, public services, transportation, and telecommunications" (National Easter Seal Society, 1990). Each of these areas is defined and discussed in later sections of this article.[1]

ADA is a broad law that affects employers, building contractors, architects, landlords, and many others (Jordan-Johnson, 1992), including those responsible for planning, administering, and implementing recreation programs and leisure time activities. The most significant areas probably will be employment issues and building modifications, with particular implications and applications to program accommodations related to recreation programs and leisure time activities.

ADA is about education, not litigation. This will help rule the success of ADA's implementation (President's Committee on Employment of People

with Disabilities, n.d.). "People really and truly want to do what is right, but sometimes it takes a law to be passed" (Jordan-Johnson, 1992, p. C2). "Where past laws dealing with civil rights tried to change attitudes and behavior, this law uniquely reaches out and physically changes the way buildings will be built and used" (Copeland, 1992, p. F1). "This ... law introduces enforceable standards ... to help persons with disabilities live mainstreamed lives as productive, contributing members of American communities" (National Easter Seal Society, 1990).

The Americans with Disabilities Act:

* Requires places of public accommodation and commercial facilities to be designed, constructed, and altered in compliance with ADA standards.
* Provides that no individual shall be discriminated against on the basis of disability in full and equal enjoyment of goods, services, facilities, privileges, advantages, or accommodations in any place of public accommodation by any private entity which owns, leases, leases to or operates a place of public accommodation.
* Stipulates places of public accommodation shall afford such goods and services in the most integrated setting appropriate to needs of individuals with disabilities (Eastern Paralyzed Veterans Association, n.d.).

For deaf, hard of hearing, blind, and partially sighted individuals, ADA will be of tremendous help in removing communication barriers in many public places. For the first time, individuals with such disabilities also have legal rights to use and fully enjoy

1. Portions of this article have been adapted and extended from *Removing Barriers in Places of Public Accommodation* (Eastern Paralyzed Veterans Association, 75-20 Astoria Blvd., Jackson Heights, NY 11370-1177).

> Note: This discussion of the ADA should not be construed as legal opinion; legal counsel should be consulted for full interpretation of the law.

public accommodations (Gallaudet University Alumni Association, 1991). "Blatant discrimination, such as prohibiting people in wheelchairs from attending movies, will be banned, along with more subtle customs such as requiring a driver's license to cash a check, which discriminates against the blind" (Copeland, 1992, p. F1).

The only two exceptions to public accommodation requirements are private clubs and religious organizations, including houses of worship and schools controlled by religious organizations (private homes and apartments are not included). However, if facilities of a private club are made available to customers or patrons of a place of public accommodation, then such facilities are covered under ADA regulations, e.g., a private club provided free or with a rental fee to a recreation department for a dance or an awards banquet. Both the landlord who owns a building housing a place of public accommodation and the tenant owning or operating the place of public accommodation are subject to ADA regulations. Determination of responsibility for complying with these regulations may be distributed by lease or other contract (Eastern Paralyzed Veterans Association, n.d.).

People with Disabilities Defined

Discrimination affects all categories of people with disabilities. Wording and interpretations of who is covered by ADA are virtually identical to Section 504 of the Rehabilitation Act, and include:

- Individuals with mobility impairments, sensory impairments, mental retardation, and other physical and mental impairments.
- Individuals who have hidden disabilities such as cancer, diabetes, epilepsy, heart disease, and mental illness, including people with HIV.
- Individuals who have a history of disability but are no longer disabled, such as a person who had, but no longer has, cancer, or a person who was misclassified as being mentally retarded.
- Individuals who do not have a disability, but who are treated or perceived by others as having a disability (Scott, 1990).

Individuals with various specified conditions are not considered to be disabled and, as such, are *not* protected against discrimination under ADA. Among

conditions excluded for ADA protection are current illegal users of drugs, homosexuals and bisexuals, and individuals with conditions such as transvestism, transsexualism, pedophilia, exhibitionism, voyeurism, gender identity disorders not resulting from physical impairments, other sexual behavior disorders, compulsive gambling, kleptomania, pyromania, and psychoactive substance use disorders resulting from current illegal use of drugs. Environmental, cultural, or economic disadvantages, such as having a prison record or being poor, are not included. Age is not considered a disability. Because the definition is so broad, it will open the door to a lot of litigation (Jordan-Johnson, 1992).

ADA—A Civil Rights Mandate

ADA is a civil rights mandate extending previous civil rights legislation—Civil Rights Act of 1964 (barring discrimination on the basis of race, creed, color, or national origin); Title IX of the Education Amendments of 1972 (barring discrimination on the basis of sex); Section 504 of the Rehabilitation Act of 1973 (barring discrimination on the basis of disability in programs operated by recipients of federal aid) — to 43 million individuals with disabilities in private sector employment and mandating equal access to public accommodations.

ADA covers:

- Employment in the private sector
- Public accommodations
- Services provided by state and local governments
- Transportation services
- Telecommunications services

ADA has been modeled after Section 504 of the Rehabilitation Act of 1973. Provisions, and in many places wording, are virtually identical to those in Section 504. Major differences between the two laws are that ADA is much more encompassing and that Section 504 applies only to programs administered by recipients of federal aid (city, municipal, and community recreation departments; city owned and operated swimming pools; public schools; colleges and universities) while ADA applies to programs in places of public accommodations, regardless of sponsor. The legislation thus applies to places of exercise and recreation, health spas, health-care providers, YM/YWCAs, YM/YWHAs, youth sport programs, gymnasiums, private swimming pools, stadiums, and arenas.

Separate But Equal Not Good Enough

"Separate, special or different programs that are designed to provide a benefit to persons with disabilities cannot be used in any way to restrict the participation of disabled persons in general integrated activities" (Judiciary Committee staff quoted in Scott, 1990, p. 17). Modified participation for individuals with disabilities is a choice, not a requirement. For example, a person without vision may choose not to participate in a special museum tour allowing people to touch sculptures in an exhibit, and instead tour the exhibit at his/her own pace with the museum's recorded tour. The Judiciary Committee staff concludes: "It is not the intent of this title to require the blind person to avail himself or herself of the special tour."

Another example is an individual with a physical condition such as spinal cord injury, amputation, or cerebral palsy wanting to be part of a regular, rather than a special segregated, arts and crafts program. To be in the regular program is the individual's right, guaranteed under ADA. The sponsor of the program is responsible for recognizing the participant's right, making necessary accommodations, and including the individual in the regular arts and crafts program.

ADA specifies that public accommodations cannot provide unequal benefits to persons with disabilities. An accommodation cannot provide a separate benefit to a person with a disability, unless the facility can show that a separate benefit is necessary to provide an opportunity to the disabled individual that is as effective as that provided to others (Scott, 1990).

A separate benefit can be justified if an individual's condition or behavior is such that learning and participation of other individuals in the program are adversely affected. Even though this separate benefit is warranted, it must be as effective as that provided others, as regards facility used, equipment and devices available, qualifications of instructors and leaders, and overall length of the program.

Places of Public Accommodation

Definitions of places of public accommodation include several categories with direct references to recreation facilities and their programs. Most other categories of public accommodation have both implications and applications for agencies and organizations operating and/or sponsoring recreation and leisure programs, whether through direct services or by extended or contract services.[2] All types of recreation and leisure facilities, programs, and activities must be interpreted in their broadest sense, including:

- Arts and crafts
- Camping and other outdoor activities, including those in wilderness areas, risk and nonrisk activities, and adventure and ropes courses
- Dramatics, drama productions, theatre, and movies
- Organized hobby programs and activities
- Outings, including hiking and picnics
- Physical activities, including physical fitness programs
- Playground and play area activities, including those involving equipment
- Rhythm and dance activities
- Social activities and outings, including field trips and visitations
- Special celebrations, including holidays and other special events
- Sports and games, including both participant and spectator roles
- Swimming and other aquatic activities
- Travel/tourism and sightseeing of all types
- Vocal and instrumental music

In all situations, individuals with disabilities must have opportunities to be active program participants, as well as to be spectators. They must have places in audiences with able-bodied families and friends at all activities, including physical, recreational, sport, and related programs.

The list of categories of establishments covered by ADA is extensive and exhaustive. Categories should be interpreted broadly since it is the intent of ADA to give people with disabilities equal access to the full range of establishments, services, and programs available to other members of society.

---

2. *The Americans with Disabilities Act: An Easy Checklist* (National Easter Seal Society, 70 East Lake St., Chicago, IL 60601) provides useful and helpful checklists for Title I—Employment and Title III—Public Accommodations and Services Operated by Private Entities.

Certain private entities are considered public accommodations under ADA if operations of such entities affect commerce. Examples of concern to recreation and physical activity personnel include:

- Motion picture houses, theatres, concert halls, stadiums, arenas, and other places of exhibition or entertainment.
- Auditoriums, convention centers, lecture halls, and other places of public gathering.
- Museums, libraries, galleries, and other places of public displays or collections.
- Parks, zoos, amusement parks, water parks, and other places of recreation.
- Nurseries; elementary, secondary, undergraduate, and postgraduate schools; and other places of education (both private and public).
- Day care centers, senior citizen centers, homeless shelters, and other social service center establishments.
- Gymnasiums, health spas, bowling alleys, golf courses, tennis courts, camps, campgrounds, and other places of exercise or recreation.

All of these places of public accommodation are required to provide auxiliary aids and services to ensure effective communication with deaf and hard of hearing people and individuals with vision impairments, including accessibility of information about programs and activities as well as physical accessibility.

The list of auxiliary aids and services required by ADA is comprehensive and includes qualified interpreters who are able to interpret effectively, accurately, and impartially both receptively and expressively, using any necessary specialized vocabulary. Other examples of auxiliary aids for deaf and hard of hearing people include notetakers, computer-assisted transcription devices, written material, telephone handset amplifiers, assistive listening devices and systems, telephones compatible with hearing aids, TDDs, video-text displays, and open and closed captioning.

Movie theatres are not required to present open-captioned films, but producers of videotapes and slide presentations are required to caption the text. The regulation also provides broad protection for use of service animals, such as guide or signal dogs or other animals trained to provide assistance to a person with a disability (Gallaudet University Alumni Association, 1991).

Readily Accessible and Readily Achievable

Interpretations by Judiciary Committee staff indicated that "the concepts 'readily accessible' and 'readily achievable' are sharply distinguishable and represent almost polar opposites in focus" (Scott, 1990). Specifically:

Readily accessible to and usable by individuals with disabilities "focuses on the person with a disability and addresses the degree of ease with which an individual with a disability can enter and use a facility; it is access and usability which must be ready" (Scott).
Readily achievable "focuses on the business operator and addresses degree of ease or difficulty of the business in removing a barrier; if barrier removal cannot be accomplished readily, then it is not required" (Scott).

Readily achievable is a basic principle built into ADA to guide barrier removal efforts in ways easily accomplishable and able to be carried out without much difficulty or expense or without undue hardship (defined as an action requiring significant difficulty or expense).

Factors to consider in determining whether an action is readily achievable or not include:

- Nature and cost of action needed.
- Overall financial resources of site(s) involved, number of persons employed at site(s), effects on expenses and resources, legitimate safety requirements necessary for safe operation including crime prevention measures, or impact of action upon operation(s) or site(s).
- Geographic separateness and administration or fiscal relationship(s) or site(s) in question to any corporation or entity.
- Overall financial resources of any parent corporation or entity; overall size of the parent corporation or entity with respect to number of its employees; and number, type, and location of its facilities.

Barrier removal measures not easily accomplishable and not able to be carried out without much difficulty or expense are not required under the "readily achievable" standard, even if they do not impose an undue burden or an undue hardship.

Examples of reasonable accommodations in various recreation and leisure time activities that are readily achievable, do not represent undue hardships on programs, and promote integration of program participants with and without disabilities include:

- Arts and crafts—provide tables that enable individuals in wheelchairs to participate fully; have adapted equipment for grasp and manipulation.
- Aquatic programs—have a buddy swim with a participant who is blind; pair individuals with and without disabilities in SCUBA instructional programs; provide aqua-stairs-ramps to assist persons in gaining access to swimming areas; use flotation devices where appropriate for individuals with severe disabilities (Reynolds, 1991).
- Dramatics and drama activities—design roles enabling individuals in wheelchairs or on gurneys to take part (e.g., bird in a gilded cage); provide a variety of opportunities, interpretive reading, for example, in addition to stage.
- Music activities—introduce and use rhythm bands where the variety of instruments allows participation for individuals with virtually any disability, especially with preschool and primary school level children; incorporate bell choirs (even removing clappers when necessary for some individuals!) for persons with various disabilities.
- Physical fitness activities—perform aerobic workouts in wheelchairs, with walkers, or on crutches; use wooden dowels or broom sticks and fishing weights of various sizes for weight training programs for individuals unable to use conventional free weights or single unit-multistation devices; devise ways in which exercise bikes (or regular bicycles supported on their handle bars and seats) can be driven with the hands and arms by individuals with lower extremity conditions; incorporate passive aerobic activities using power driven apparatus for individuals with extremely severe and/or profound conditions.
- Rhythm and dance activities—slow records down; provide opportunities for individuals with hearing impairments to get the beat by touching a speaker, feeling vibrations through a balloon, wooden floor, or other objects in the room, especially when volume is increased over usual levels; use partners as necessary and appropriate, regardless of disability; encourage participants in wheelchairs, with walkers, or on crutches to respond to movement commands in their own ways.
- Sports and games—participate fully while wearing arm/hand or leg/foot prosthetic devices (individuals with various types and degrees of amputations); use guide runners, tethers, and other assistive devices in distance running, road races, and marathons (runners who are blind or with various visual impairments); encourage different assistive devices such as ramps, pushers, special handle balls for bowling (participants with conditions such as spinal cord injuries, amputations, cerebral palsy); adjust position of starter's gun (down rather than up) in track and swimming races (competitors who are deaf or hard of hearing).

Regulations Governing Public Accommodations

Specific provisions of ADA and its rules and regulations governing public accommodations are requirements to:

- Make reasonable changes in policies, practices, and procedures to avoid participant discrimination (e.g., not requiring physical/medical examinations of individuals with disabilities if such examinations are not required of all program participants).
- Provide auxiliary aids and services to individuals with vision or hearing impairments or other individuals with disabilities so they can have equal opportunities to participate or benefit, unless an undue burden would result (e.g., use brightly colored balls so individuals with visual impairments can participate in games such as volleyball; use some type of conventional signs to communicate with program participants having hearing impairments).
- Remove physical barriers in existing facilities if removal is readily achievable (e.g., provide ramps, make curb cuts, increase number of parking spaces for persons with disabilities). If not, alternative methods of providing the services must be offered, if those methods are readily achievable (e.g., use portable or temporary ramps or inexpensive chair lifts or terrace out steps altogether).
- Make accessible all new construction in public accommodations, as well as in commercial facilities (such as office buildings), including recreation facilities such as gymnasiums, arenas, health spas, and bowling alleys.
- Be sure alterations are accessible. When alterations to primary function areas are made, an accessible path of travel to the altered area—including bathrooms, telephones, and drinking fountains—must be provided to the extent that added accessibility costs are not disproportionate to overall cost of alterations (U.S. Department of Justice, 1990).

Design Specifications

ADA regulations contain a wide ranging list of modest and readily achievable measures that may be taken to remove barriers. Examples of such measures include, but are not limited to, installing ramps, making curb cuts in sidewalks and entrances; repositioning shelves; rearranging tables, chairs, vending machines, and other funiture; repositioning telephones and using long cords for handsets; adding braille or raised markings on elevator control buttons, having elevators speak electronically, and installing inexpensive and easily positioned pointers to engage floor selectors for individuals unable to reach regular floor selectors; installing flashing alarm lights; widening doors, installing offset hinges to widen doorways, eliminating turnstiles or providing alternative accessible paths; installing accessible door hardware, installing grab bars in toilet stalls, rearranging toilet partitions to increase maneuvering space; creating designated accessible parking spaces; installing an accessible paper cup dispenser at an existing drinking fountain.

For detailed discussion and elaboration of each of these and other measures, see *Removing Barriers in Places of Public Accommodation* (Eastern Paralyzed Veterans Association).

Accessibility—
Practical Considerations

ADA regulations contain basic design specifications for making a variety of building elements and fixtures more accessible to and usable by individuals with disabilities. Representative examples of both general and specific measures expected to make facilities and programs accessible include:

- Make it possible for individuals to get through doors and have actual physical access to a facility from public sidewalks, public transportation, or parking by installing ramps or wheelchair platform lifts, widening entrances, and providing accessible parking spaces.
- Maintain in operable working condition features of facilities and equipment required for ready accessibility to and use by persons with disabilities.
- Provide access to areas of public accommodation where goods and services are made available to the public by adjusting layout of display racks, rearranging tables, providing braille and raised character signs, widening doors, using visual alarms, and installing ramps.
- Provide a reasonable number of wheelchair seating places and removable aisle-side armrests. Locate wheelchair seating places so they are distributed throughout the seating area; provide line of sight vision and choice of admission prices comparable to those for members of the general public; have an accessible route that also serves as a means of egress in case of an emergency; permit individuals who

use wheelchairs to sit with family members and other companions.
- Provide access to restroom facilities. If separate restroom facilities for each sex are provided, then each should be rendered accessible if readily achievable. However, accessible unisex restroom facilities are acceptable.
- Take any other measures necessary to provide access to goods, services, facilities, privileges, advantages, or accommodations of a place of public accommodation. Representative examples of such measures include:
  — making at least one loading zone accessible (e.g., providing an access aisle which is at least 20 feet long and 5 feet wide and equipped with a curb ramp);
  — relocating operable controls to acceptable reach ranges of persons with disabilities (at a height of 48 inches from the finished floor if a forward approach is intended or 54 inches if a side approach is necessary);
  — identifying accessible facilities with the international symbol of accessibility;
  — having thresholds at doors beveled and no higher than 3/4 inch;
  — providing easily operable faucet controls for lavatory and faucet access.

For detailed discussion and elaboration of these and other similar measures, see *Removing Barriers in Places of Public Accommodation* (Eastern Paralyzed Veterans Association, p. 14-24).

Specific Applications to Recreation and Related Facilities

Final regulations indicate places of public accommodation such as health-care providers, service establishments, places of recreation, gymnasiums, health spas, and other places of exercise or recreation can take into consideration safety criteria, and may "impose neutral rules and criteria that screen out, or tend to screen out, individuals with disabilities, if the criteria are necessary for the safe operation of the public accommodation." Examples of safety qualifications that would be justifiable in appropriate circumstances would include a height requirement for certain amusement park rides or the requirement that all participants in a recreational rafting expedition be able to meet a necessary swimming proficiency. Safety requirements must be based on actual risks and not on speculation, stereotypes, or generalizations about individual disabilities (*Federal Register* 56, No. 144, p. 35564, July 26, 1991).

The regulations also indicate that where an individual poses a direct threat to health or safety of others, a place of public accommodation is not required to permit an individual to participate in or benefit from its goods, services, facilities, privileges, advantages, and accommodations. Under the comments to this rule, however, "A public accommodation is required to make an individualized assessment, based on reasonable judgment that relies on the best available objective evidence to determine: the nature, duration, severity of the risk; the probability that potential injury will actually occur; and whether reasonable modifications of policies, practices, or procedures will mitigate the risk" (*Federal Register* 56, No. 144, p. 35560, July 26, 1991). Therefore, health and fitness facilities may need to revise operational policies to ensure that services are available to individuals with disabilities (Herbert, 1991b).

Historic Properties and Wilderness Areas

Several provisions of ADA are directly related and applicable to qualified historic properties and federal wilderness areas. Specifically:

Qualified historic properties—ADA requires supplemental guidelines to incorporate standards developed under the Uniform Federal Accessibility Standards (UFAS) for qualified historic buildings undergoing alterations. These standards should ensure that qualified historic structures are not altered in such a manner that would threaten or destroy their historical significance (Scott, 1990).

Colonial Williamsburg (Virginia) is an excellent example of a historic site which, even prior to ADA, has been sensitive and responsive to special needs of visitors with various disabilities (Colonial Williamsburg). Although Colonial Williamsburg is largely accessible and staff members are prepared to make special accommodations when necessary, services are continually being evaluated to determine ways in which the historic area can be even more accessible. Representative of special services enabling visitors with disabilities to participate in and enjoy this historic site of 18th-century architecture are:

- Visitors with visual impairments—licensed guide dogs are permitted in all buildings; special tours can be arranged; hands-on activities are permitted at certain exhibitions.
- Visitors with hearing impairments—a special brochure, *Colonial Williamsburg: A Guide for Deaf and Hearing Impaired Visitors,* is designed to enhance Williamsburg experiences for visitors with hearing impairments. A printed synopsis of the orientation film, *Williamsburg—The Story of a Patriot,* is available, as are special headsets with adjustable volume controls. With advanced notice, a special screening of the captioned version of the film may be scheduled. Colonial Williamsburg has several signing interpreters available to accompany visitors with hearing impairments through the historic area.
- Visitors with limited mobility—streets, most gardens, and outdoor activities of the historic area are easily accessible to individuals in wheelchairs. A special *Wheelchair Guide* provides detailed information about accessibility to visitors in wheelchairs of all exhibitions and buildings. While portable ramps are available at selected exhibitions, nearly all buildings require at least a few steps. Many of the exhibition buildings have second floors requiring negotiating steps that are often steep and narrow. Some buildings are featured in special audiovisual presentations that interpret their second floors so visitors can avoid negotiating the stairs.

Collapsible wheelchairs can be taken on busses going from the visitor center to the historic areas. Although electric wheelchairs and electric scooters are not now permitted on existing busses, plans include expanding the transportation system so visitors with electric mobility devices can be accommodated.

Federal wilderness areas—Under ADA, no individual with a disability may be discriminated against with respect to entrance to wilderness areas. The law stipulates that wheelchairs[3] may be used in wilderness areas notwithstanding a provision in the Wilderness Act that prohibits "motorized equipment and other mechanical transport" within wilderness areas. However, "no agency is required to provide any form of special treatment or accommodation, or to construct any facilities or modify any conditions of lands within a wilderness area in order to facilitate such use" (U.S. House of Representatives, 1990, Sec. 507(c)(1)).

––––––––––

3. Wheelchair is defined as a device designed solely for use by a mobility-impaired person for locomotion that is suitable for use in an indoor pedestrian area.

Additional ADA Requirements

ADA also includes requirements for employment, transportation, state and local government operations, and telecommunications.

Employment

No covered entity shall discriminate against a qualified individual with a disability because of a disability in regard to job application procedures, hiring, advancement, employee compensation, job training, and other privileges. Employers may not discriminate in hiring or promoting an individual with a disability who is otherwise qualified for the position. Employers need to provide reasonable accommodations to qualified applicants or employees with disabilities, including steps such as job restructuring and modifying equipment.

Establishments involved in any aspect of recreation, leisure, and related services must comply with the regulations and can in no way discriminate against individuals with disabilities who are otherwise qualified for positions in their programs. A case in point is a July 1992 court order enabling a paraplegic in a wheelchair to continue coaching baseball, despite a Little League rule barring his wheelchair from the field. A Phoenix, Arizona, judge ruled that prohibiting this individual to coach behind third base was a violation of ADA (Associated Press, 1992c).

ADA requirements regarding employment—and applicable to all types of organizations and agencies providing physical, recreational, leisure, and sport activities—include:

- Remove physical and communication barriers.
- Provide reasonable accommodations, such as special equipment, interpreters, or flexible working hours.
- Remove job application questions on illnesses, injuries, disabilities, and worker's compensation claims.
- Remove unrelated physical requirements from job descriptions.
- Limit medical examination reports to job related concerns (Associated Press, 1992b).

Transportation

No qualified individual with a disability shall be excluded from participation in or be denied benefits of services, programs, or activities of public entities, including transportation. A public accommodation that provides transportation services, even though such services are not their primary business, must remove transportation barriers to persons with disabilities. Examples of such services include:

- Vans and busses operated by camps and community recreation agencies.
- Student transportation systems.
- Transportation provided within recreational facilities such as stadiums, zoos, parks, and ski resorts.

Places of public accommodation in such situations are urged to follow required terminal design standards and vehicle specifications prepared by the Architectural and Transportation Barriers Compliance Board (Eastern Paralyzed Veterans Association).

An unanswered question at the time this was written involves responsibility of a recreation department or camp to provide transportation to participants with disabilities. Obviously, if transportation is provided individuals without disabilities, then accessible transportation must be provided individuals with disabilities. The response is not clearcut if transportation is not provided individuals without disabilities. Although such situations are dealt with under Individuals with Disabilities Education Act (IDEA, formerly Education of All Handicapped Children Act, P.L. 94-142), similar precedents cannot be found under Section 504 of the Rehabilitation Act. Only time and results of litigation will provide a definitive answer to this question.

State and Local Government Operations

ADA directly addresses and impacts services, activities, and programs of state and local governments, extending and reinforcing provisions of Section 504 of the Rehabilitation Act of 1973. Specifically:

- State and local governments may not discriminate against qualified individuals with disabilities (parks and recreation departments are arms of state and local governments).
- All government facilities, services, and communications must be accessible, consistent with requirements of Section 504 of the Rehabilitation Act (U.S. Department of Justice, 1990a, 1990c).

Telecommunications

ADA amends Title II of the Communications Act of 1934 by adding a section providing that the Federal Communications Commission ensured interstate and intrastate telecommunications relay services must be available, to the extent possible, to individuals with hearing and speech impairments. Specifically, companies offering telephone service to the general public must offer telephone relay service to individuals who use telecommunications devices for the deaf (TDDs) or similar devices (U.S. Department of Justice, 1990a, 1990c).

ADA requires that all television public service announcements produced or financed, in whole or part, by federal funding must include closed captioning to permit hearing impaired people to read verbal contents of the announcements. Regular closed captioning must be provided by producers, not broadcasters, of programs receiving federal assistance.

Some Practical Steps for Implementing ADA

Full impact of compliance with ADA regulations has not been fully felt yet, but will have significant impact on financial planning and personnel selection and development. Practical advice includes:

- Set up an advisory committee including persons with disabilities. Draw on other resources such as families, social professionals, educators, and the medical and business communities.
- Review current program protocols in line with regulations, looking for questionable practices.
- Educate staff, including boards and CEOs, about ADA through preservice and inservice training.
- Train staff to eliminate discriminatory remarks from their vocabularies and heighten their awareness about cost of litigation resulting from inappropriate comments (see National Easter Seal Society, *Tips for Disability Awareness* and *Tips for Portraying People with Disabilities in the Media* for practical assistance in these areas).
- Extend practical experience opportunities to staff in use of communication aids, sign language, wheelchairs, prosthetic devices, lifts, and transfers.
- Review current program applications, health care statement forms, and other documents to ensure that the language does not discriminate in any way.
- If you are asked about accessibility of your program by a person whose disability you are not sure can be accommodated, seek advice before responding (Reynolds, 1991).
- Review safety considerations and procedures to assure that individuals with disabilities can take part safely or legitimately be denied access to hazardous situations.

Enforcement

The employment section of ADA incorporates powers, remedies, and procedures set forth in Title VII of the Civil Rights Act of 1964. These remedies include injunctive relief, back pay, and attorney's fees (Scott, 1990). Enforcement of ADA employment provisions is by the Equal Employment Opportunity Commission, 1801 L St., NW, Washington, DC 20507, voice—202-663-4900; TDD—800-800-3302.

The public accommodations section of ADA provides the same enforcement procedures and remedies as under Title III of the Civil Rights Act for individuals with disabilities who are subject to discrimination by public accommodations. However, remedies are restricted to injunctive relief such as an injunction to require a public accommodation to undertake a readily achievable barrier removal.

In addition to private lawsuits brought by individuals with disabilities, the public accommodations section of ADA authorizes the Justice Department to bring action against a pattern or practice of discrimination. ADA also provides that an action for injunctive relief can be brought by any person who has reasonable grounds for believing that construction of a new building, or alterations to an existing building, are about to begin that would not provide access to those with disabilities (Scott, 1990).

Enforcement of ADA public accommodation provisions is by the Department of Justice (Coordination and Review Section, Civil Rights Division, P.O. Box 66118, Washington, DC 20035-6118, voice—202-514-0381; TDD—202-514-0381/83.

Transit authorities failing to implement ADA requirements may be considered to have discriminated against people with disabilities and may be sued for injunctive relief under Sections 504 and 505 of the Rehabilitation Act of 1973 (Scott, 1990). Enforcement of ADA transportation provisions is by the Department of Transportation, 400 Seventh St., SW, Washington, DC 20509, voice—202-366-9305; TDD—202-755-7687.

In general, enforcement of telephone relay requirements is carried out through existing enforcement provisions of the Communications Act of 1934. Enforcement of ADA telecommunications provisions is by the Federal Communications Commission, 1919 M St., NW, Washington, DC 20554, voice—202-632-7260; TDD—202-632-6999.

A Challenge to All

George Bush, as president of the United States, at a commemorative celebration in the Rose Garden of the White House, summed up the work of educating the nation on ADA:

"We have worked together this last year, and in so doing, we've understood more fully just how much people with disabilities have to offer. We've demonstrated that social progress includes economic growth—and that both play essential roles in the American dream. Businesses support the ADA because it gives everyone a chance to be productive in the workplace. It broadens our economic mainstream. It enables society to benefit from the wisdom, energy and industry of people who want just one thing—a fair chance.

"And while we've made a strong start, we have much to do. As long as the doors of opportunity are closed to even one American—we must keep working at it."

Essential to compliance is a thorough understanding of ADA intent and requirements and an ongoing commitment to understanding needs and rights of individuals with disabilities, regardless of type or severity of such conditions. Necessary facility accessibility, appropriate program accommodations, positive participant and leader attitudes, and ongoing advocacy must be our guiding lights to equal opportunities and excellence of results.

And, until every American—regardless of age, type and severity of disability, background, and experience—has opportunities to be an active participant in physical activity, physical education, recreation and leisure time, sport, dance, and related programs, we must accept this as our professional challenge and personal goal and keep working to make the dream our reality.

Selected References and Resources

Associated Press. (1992a). Firms required to strip barriers to disabled. *Knoxville News-Sentinel*, July 26, 1992, p. A6.

Associated Press. (1992b). Requirements of Disabilities Act. *Knoxville News-Sentinel*, July 26, 1992, p. A6.

Associated Press. (1992c). Paraplegic can coach. *Oak Ridger*, July 9, 1992, p. 10.

Colonial Williamsburg: A guide for visitors with disabilities. Williamsburg, VA: Colonial Williamsburg Foundation (Visitor Services Coordinator).

Colonial Williamsburg: Wheelchair guide. Williamsburg, VA: Colonial Williamsburg Foundation (Visitor Services Coordinator).

Copeland, Peter. (1992). Breaking the barriers: Disabilities Act will change shape of U.S. buildings. *Knoxville News-Sentinel*, January 12, 1992, p. F1, 5.

Eastern Paralyzed Veterans Association. *Removing barriers in places of public accommodation.* Jackson Heights, NY: Eastern Paralyzed Veterans Association (75-20 Astoria Blvd., 11370-1177).

Equal Employment Opportunity Commission, 1801 L St., NW, Washington, DC 20507. Most publications are available in accessible formats such as braille, large print, audiotape, and electronic file on computer disk:
Americans with Disabilities Act: Your responsibilities as an employer — question and answer format; available in English and Spanish, 17 pp.
Americans with Disabilities Act: Your employment rights as an individual with a disability — available in English and Spanish, 11 pp.
Information for the private sector and state and local governments.

Gallaudet University Alumni Association. (1991). Final ADA regulations issued by Justice Department. *Gallaudet Alumni Newsletter*, 26 (2), 1.

Goldman, Charles D. (1991). *Disability rights guide* (2nd ed.). Lincoln, NE: Media Publishing (2440 O St., Suite 202, 68510).

Herbert, David L. (1991a). The Americans with Disabilities Act. *Fitness Management*, 7 (4), 32-36.

Herbert, David L. (1991b). Update on the Americans with Disabilities Act. *Fitness Management*, 7 (11), October, 30-31.

Jordan-Johnson, Stephanie. (1992). Workplace: New law bars employers from discriminating against the disabled. *Washington Post*, June 7, 1992, C2.

McGovern, John. (1992) *ADA self-evaluation handbook and checklist* (1st ed.). (Designed especially for city and county park and recreation departments and other leisure service agencies.) Arlington, VA: National Recreation and Park Association (2775 S. Quincy St., Suite 300, 22206).

National Easter Seal Society, 70 East Lake St., Chicago, IL 60601:
    Awareness is the first step brochures: The Americans with Disabilities Act; Tips for disability awareness; Tips for portraying people with disabilities in the media; The Fair Housing Amendments Act; The Air Carrier Access Act (40 cents each).
    Nobody is burning wheelchairs — 15 min. videotape showing contributions of individuals with disabilities as qualified and competent employees working toward total integration in a completely accessible society ($35, 1/2" VHS or 3/3", both with and without open captioning).
    Part of the team — 17 min. videotape profiling successful working relations between employers and their employees with disabilities ($15, 1/2" VHS; $25, 3/4", both with and without open captioning).
    The Americans with Disabilities Act: An easy checklist (1990) — 14-page booklet designed to help businesses evaluated current policies and procedures for meeting ADA requirements ($1.00).
    The workplace workbook — an illustrated guide to job accommodations and assistive technology ($32).

President's Committee on Employment of People with Disabilities. ADA anniversary celebration, President's Committee's ADA Teleconferencing Project identifies major needs and trends, and They came to Dallas. President's Committee on Employment of People with Disabilities *Newsbrief,* I (1), 5.

Reed, Vita. (1992a). Complying with Disabilities Act won't be costly, advocates say. *Knoxville News-Sentinel,* Feb. 2, 1992, D1, 3.

Reed, Vita. (1992b). New law's impact is far reaching. *Knoxville News-Sentinel,* Feb. 2, 1992, DI, 2.

Reynolds, Grace D. (1991). *Legislation and aquatics: Practical advice.* Unpublished paper. Longview, WA: Disability International Foundation (Box 1781, 98632).

Ross, Sonya. (1992). Disability Act's next phase removes hiring, physical barriers today. *Oak Ridger,* July 26, 1992, 8A.

Scott, Kimberly (Ed.). (1990). *The Americans with Disabilities Act: An analysis.* Silver Spring, MD: Business Publishers, Inc. (951 Pershing Dr., 20910-4464).

U.S. Department of Justice. (1990a). *Americans with Disabilities Act requirements fact sheet.* Washington, DC: U.S. Department of Justice (Civil Rights Division, Coordination and Review Section, P.O. Box 66118, 20035-6118). Available in braille, large print, audiotape, electronic file on computer disk, and electronic bulletin board.

U.S. Department of Justice. (1990b). Technical assistance plan for the American with Disabilities Act of 1990. *Federal Register,* 55 (234) (December 5), 50237-50249.

U.S. Department of Justice. (1990c). *The Americans with Disabilities Act.* Washington, DC: U.S. Department of Justice (Civil Rights Division, Coordination and Review Section, P.O. Box 66118, 20035-6118). Available in braille, large print, audiotape, electronic file on computer disk, and electronic bulletin board.

U.S. Department of Justice. (1991). Americans with Disabilities Act: Final rule and section by section analysis and response top comments. *Federal Register,* 57 (144), July 26.

U.S. Department of Transportation. (1991). Transportation for individuals with disabilities: Final rule. *Federal Register* (49 CFR Parts 27, 37, 38), 56 (173), Sept. 6, 45584-45777.

Ward, Hugh. (1992). The common law: The American with Disabilities Act explained. *Oak Ridger,* July 1, p. 10.

U.S. House of Representatives. (1990). Americans with Disabilities act of 1990: Conference Report, 101st Congress, 2nd Session, Report 101-596, July 12.

Legal Concerns:
Civil Rights and Negligence

Annie Clement

The legal areas of greatest concern to play-ground professionals working with individuals with disabilities are civil rights and negligence. In this article discussion of civil rights or rights of participants will focus primarily on the Americans with Disabilities Act of 1990 (Public Law No. 101-366, 104 Stat. 327, July 26, 1990) and will briefly review earlier legislation. Negligence will be defined and discussed in the context of appropriate standards of care. A system of risk management, tailored to meet the rights of participants, and negligence is provided.

Rights of the Participant

Most civil rights law is attached in some way to the 14th Amendment to the Constitution. To better understand the rights of participants, the reader should examine the following portion of the 14th Amendment. "No state shall make or enforce any law which shall abridge the privileges or immunities of citizens of the United States; nor shall any state deprive any person of life, liberty, or property, without due process of law; nor deny to any person within its jurisdiction the equal protection of the law."

The equal protection clause establishes that all people are equal and are expected to be treated as equals. The Americans with Disabilities Act of 1990 describes what that treatment should be.

The Act became effective January 1992 and all aspects of the legislation were in effect by summer 1992. Although the Americans with Disabilities Act

is considered to be more stringent than most state laws, professionals are to be aware of and to adhere to state law.

Americans with Disabilities Act

The purpose of the Americans with Disabilities Act of 1990 (ADA) is to:

(1) provide a clear and comprehensive national mandate for the elimination of discrimination against individuals with disabilities;
(2) provide clear, strong, consistent, enforceable standards addressing discrimination against individuals with disabilities;
(3) ensure that the Federal Government plays a central role in enforcing the standards established in this Act on behalf of individuals with disabilities; and
(4) invoke the sweep of congressional authority, including the power to enforce the fourteenth amendment and to regulate commerce, in order to address the major areas of discrimination faced day-to-day by people with disabilities" (ADA, Sec. 2[b]).

Although considerable legislation with reference to disabilities exists, until ADA there has not been a comprehensive approach to providing for the needs of the disabled. Through ADA, Congress has given the federal government a mandate to eliminate discrimination against persons with disabilities and the power to enforce the mandate.

The term "disability," for the purpose of the Act, means, with respect to an individual:

(A) a physical or mental impairment that substantially limits one or more of the major life activities of such individuals;
(B) a record of such an impairment; or
(C) being regarded as having such an impairment (ADA, Sec. 3[2]).

Title III of the Act, Public Accommodations and Services Operated by Private Entities, Section 301, No. 7, I through L, specifically covers areas used as playgrounds. They are:

(I) a park, zoo, amusement park, or other place of recreation;
(J) a nursery, elementary, secondary, undergraduate, or postgraduate private school, or other place of education;
(K) a day care center, senior citizen center, homeless shelter, food bank, adoption agency or other social service center establishment, and
(L) a gymnasium, health spa, bowling alley, golf course, or other place of exercise or recreation.

Playgrounds, indoors and outdoors, park, recreation, or school, and forms of amusement that might be considered playgrounds are controlled by the Act.

As the Act goes into effect a key phrase in the law, "readily achievable," will receive attention. According to ADA "readily achievable" means "easily accomplishable and able to be carried out without much difficulty or expense." In determining whether an action is readily achievable, factors to be considered include:

(A) the nature and cost of the action needed under this Act;
(B) the overall financial resources of the facility or facilities involved in the action; the number of persons employed at such facility; the effect on expenses and resources, or the impact otherwise of such action upon the operation of the facility;
(C) the overall financial resources of the covered entity; the overall size of the business of a covered entity with respect to the number of its employees; the number, type, and location of its facilities; and
(D) the type of operation or operations of the covered entity, including the composition, structure, and functions of the work force of such entity; the geographic separateness, administrative or fiscal relationship of the facility or facilities in question to the covered entity (ADA, Sec. 301 [9]).

Although the above phrase appears to support those who do not want to change, further reading of the law establishes that it will be enforced. For example, note the specific prohibitions of discrimination under construction:

(i) the imposition or application of eligibility criteria that screen out or tend to screen out an individual with a disability or any class of individuals with disabilities from fully and equally enjoying any goods, services, facilities, privileges, advantages, or accommodations, unless such criteria can be shown to be necessary for the provision of the goods, services, facilities, privileges, advantages, or accommodations being offered;
(ii) a failure to make reasonable modifications in policies, practices, or procedures, when such modifications are necessary to afford such goods, services, facilities, privileges, advantages, or accommodations to individuals with disabilities, unless the entity can demonstrate that making such modifications would fundamentally alter the nature of such goods, services, facilities, privileges, advantages, or accommodations;
(iii) a failure to take such steps as may be necessary to ensure that no individual with a disability is excluded, denied services, segregated or otherwise treated differently than other individuals because of the absence of auxiliary aids and services, unless the entity can demonstrate that taking such steps would fundamentally alter the nature of the good, service, facility, privilege, advantage, or accommodation being offered or would result in an undue burden;
(iv) a failure to remove architectural barriers, and communication barriers that are structural in nature, in existing facilities, and transportation barriers in existing vehicles and rail passenger cars used by an establishment for transporting individuals (not including barriers that can only be removed through the retrofitting of vehicles or rail passenger cars by the installation of a hydraulic or other lift), where such removal is readily achievable; and
(v) where an entity can demonstrate that the removal of a barrier under clause (iv) is not readily achievable, a failure to make such goods, services, facilities, privileges, or accommodations available through alternative methods if such methods are readily achievable" (ADA, Sec. 302, [b] [2] [A]).

New facilities and those undergoing extensive remodeling within 30 months of the enactment of the law are expected to immediately conform with the law (ADA, Sec. 303, [a] [1] and [2]).

Enforcement

The Act will be enforced by the Attorney General of the United States with the following authority of the Court in civil actions:

(A) may grant any equitable relief that such court considers to be appropriate, including, to the extent required by this title:
   (i) granting temporary, preliminary, or permanent relief;
   (ii) providing an auxiliary aid or service, modification of policy, practice, or procedure, or alternative method; and
   (iii) making facilities readily accessible to and usable by individuals with disabilities;
(B) may award such other relief as the court considers to be appropriate, including monetary damages to persons aggrieved when requested by Attorney General; and
(C) may, to vindicate the public interest, assess a civil penalty against the entity in an amount:
   (i) not exceeding $50,000 for a first violation; and
   (ii) not exceeding $100,000 for any subsequent violation (ADA, sec. 308, [b] [2]).

Thus an individual or a group of individuals can bring an action to a court of law that could result in:

I. the court finding the defendant operating within the parameters of the law.
II. the court finding the defendant in violation of the law and granting:
   (a) an injunction or a demand that the activity violating the plaintiff's civil rights be stopped.
   (b) a demand that modifications be made or
   (c) a demand of modification accompanied by money damages. These money damages are assessed to assist the aggrieved individual and to assure the public that those afflicting such harm are punished.

Although implementation details of the Americans with Disabilities Act will become apparent as a result of litigation, there are examples one can envision as implementation of the law. New or renovated playgrounds are to be planned with the needs of children with disabilities in mind. For example, equipment designed for development of arm strength without the need for either balance or strength from the legs is an example of an accommodation. When a piece of equipment cannot be redesigned for a particular condition, auxiliary services are to be available. Amusement parks may choose to assist a person to a seat in a ride rather than making the ride seat wheelchair accessible. Architectural barriers in entrances, bathrooms, ramps, and curbs are eliminated in planning.

Early Legislation

The need for legislation to assist individuals with disabilities became apparent in the 1960s; however, specific legislation did not exist until the 1970s. Two cases, Pennsylvania Association for Retarded Children v. Commonwealth of Pennsylvania (1971) and Mills v. Board of Education of the District of Columbia (1972) are credited with setting standards for early legislation. Both suits were class action (groups of people); the disability in both cases was mental retardation and/or behavior problems.

The early legislation provided "a free public education which emphasizes special education and related services designed to meet their unique needs, to assure that the rights of handicapped children and their parents or guardians are protected, to assist States and localities to provide for the education of all handicapped children, and to assess and assure the effectiveness of efforts to educate handicapped children" (20 U.S.C.A. 1401).

As a result of Public Law 94-142 all children with disabilities, from age 3 to 21, receive free appropriate public education and individualized education programs (IEPs) are designed for each participant. Public Law 99-457, which took effect in 1991, and its antecedent Public Law 98-199 extends the legislation to the three to five year old and provides state grants for infants up to two years of age. The Americans with Disabilities Act extends the rights of individuals with disabilities beyond the school to all facets of life including recreation and leisure.

IEPs or school programs are designed with the special needs of each child in mind, and the unique characteristics of individuals with disabilities are accommodated in the education program. Under ADA the same thinking and planning will be extended to recreation and sport programs. Playground free space and equipment will be planned to provide for special populations.

Negligence

A second area of concern to the playground professional is negligence. Negligence is "an omission to do something which a reasonable [person] guided by those ordinary considerations which ordinarily regulate human affairs would do, or the doing of something which a reasonable and prudent [person] would not do" (*Black's Law Dictionary*).

The elements of negligence are:

- A legal duty of care.
- Breach or failure to assume that duty.
- Breach or failure is the direct cause of the injury.
- Substantial damage.

Elements of Negligence

In general, playground professionals have a legal duty of care to persons who enjoy the playground. That duty is expressed as a standard of care or standard of behavior expected of the professional. Standards for playgrounds are hypothetical and are somewhat unique to individual playgrounds. They are influenced by statutes, ordinances, administrative rules, contracts, and judicial decisions or the results of court cases. This section will assist professionals in arriving at a viable standard of care for their playground.

When a professional is sued under negligence, the person filing the suit or complaint identifies the legal duty they believe is required of the professional, alleges or proves that the legal duty was breached and that the breach was directly related to the injury. The defendant/professional responds by identifying the legal duty, admitting breach or providing evidence to support the fact that the legal duty/standard of care was adhered to, and identifies the relationship of the breach to the legal duty. The following discussion will, hopefully, impress upon the playground professional the importance of understanding and executing a standard of care that is acceptable to self and to the profession.

For example, a school's standard of playground supervision may be one teacher for every 50 students, with daily inspection. A child falls, sustaining serious injury as a result of a broken ladder on a slide. Legal duty is a combination of what a reasonable school district should do and the school's standard of supervision and inspection.

Was the legal duty breached? An investigation of the events of the day establishes that the slide ladder had not been inspected on the day of the accident and that the teacher supervising the 20 children on the playground witnessed the injury. The child sustained a serious injury or substantial damage.

Was the accident a direct result of the breach? Examination of all details by the court and/or the jury will determine the relationship.

Decision of the Court

The results of the court's decision may be:

- The defendant is found not negligent.
- The defendant is found negligent and the following damages are awarded:
  — compensatory, or restoring the plaintiff to where they were prior to the injury.
  — compensatory and, on occasion, punitive, an award designed to deter the wrong doer from continuing the behavior.

Defenses

Two defenses to negligence are contributory negligence and assumption of risk. Contributory negligence is found when injured persons are responsible, in part, for their injuries. For example, a child who is injured in falling from a swing after standing up or jumping from the equipment will be considered to have contributed to the injury. Standing or jumping from a moving swing is not an acceptable means of using that piece of equipment.

Assumption of risk means the injured party was fully aware of the risks involved and assumed the risk. Evidence or proof of the victim's assumption of risk must be provided to the court.

Comparative Negligence

Comparative negligence is a legal theory in use in many states. The cost of the injury is determined, and the fault is allocated by percentages.

For example, a plaintiff or person bringing the case may be found 20% liable or contributory negligent while the defendant may be 80% liable. A $100,000 injury or court judgment will find the plaintiff responsible for $20,000 and the defendant responsible for $80,000. Professionals preparing risk management programs will be sensitive to eliminating the chance of being even 5% or 10% liable.

Role of Playground Professionals

The major legal theories, civil rights and negligence, affecting playground professionals have been identified. Playground professionals can assume that when individuals with whom they work are denied access to equipment and/or programs or when those individuals sustain injury, they may file a legal complaint against the agency and/or its employees. Thus, playground professionals can be sued.

A playground professional should feel secure that civil rights and standards of care within their playgrounds are reasonable and meet peer scrutiny. In addition, a system for documenting the existence of individual rights and substantiating an appropriate standard of care should be followed. This system will be used to prove that the playground participant's civil rights were met and there was no way an injury could have been foreseen. Further, professionals must believe most competent colleagues would agree with the approach.

Risk Management Plan

Creation and execution of an operating civil rights procedure and an appropriate standard of care are components of a risk management plan. Playground administrators, in conjunction with their personnel, are charged with creating such a plan. Guidance for the civil rights components of the plan will come from the Americans with Disabilities Act of 1990 and other civil rights legislation, particularly those applying to individuals with disabilities. Ideas for planning with reference to negligence involve the efficient and safe use of playground space and equipment, safety in designing and building play areas, provision for adequate instruction, and attention to the results of injury statistics and litigation. Detailed information is available to guide professionals in the area of negligence, but to date only a limited amount of information is available on civil rights. Playground professionals will need to test their civil rights plans against results of court cases to be assured of their viability.

Establish Standards

Locate existing standards of playground civil rights and safety or standards of care. In addition to chapters in this book, consult the following documents:

Civil Rights

Public Law 101-366, Americans with Disabilities Act of 1990

Public Law 99-457, Education of the Handicapped Amendment Act of 1986

Public Law 98-199, Education of the Handicapped Amendment Act of 1983

Public Law 94-142, Education of Handicapped Children, 20 U.S.C.A. 1400-1461

Rehabilitation Act of 1973, 29 U.S.C. 701

Rehabilitation Act of 1973, 29 U.S.C. 504 794

Standard of Care

ASTM Standards for playground surfaces

ASTM Standards for public use of playground equipment (anticipated publication 1993)

Bauer, Eugene G., & Ronald Pinegar. (1987). *The primer for playground safety.* Grinnell, IA: Ashley Scott & Assoc.

Bruya, L.D., & Langendorfer, S.J. (Eds.). (1988). *Where our children play: Elementary school playground equipment.* Reston, VA: AAHPERD.

Moore, Robin C. (1987). *Play for all.* Berkeley, CA: MIG Communications.

Thompson, D., & Bowers, L. (Eds.). (1989). *Where our children play: Community park playground equipment.* Reston, VA: AAHPERD.

United States Consumer Product Safety Commission. (1991). *Handbook for public playground safety.* Washington, DC: U.S. Government Printing Office.

Wortham, S.C., & Frost, J.D. (Eds.). (1990). *Playgrounds for young children: National survey and perspective.* Reston, VA: AAHPERD.

Devise a theoretical statement of standards applicable for a playground with equipment and play spaces similar to that found on your playground. These standards are to be reasonable or adequate; they do not have to be perfect.

For each piece of equipment and play space provide the appropriate standard for:

- Design and construction
- Maintenance and general condition
- Age or size of participants
- Number of participants
- Skill level of participants
- Instruction
  - Is instruction needed?
  - If so, how will it be presented?
  - Printed and posted or live instruction?
  - By whom?
- Have bilingual, blind, and retarded participants' needs been met in instruction?

Using the same materials, create standards for crowd control, supervision, and injury surveillance. They should address amount of space between pieces of equipment and flow of traffic from one area to another.

Practical Application of Theoretical Standard

Structure the theoretical standard into a series of questions or a check sheet that can be used as an assessment tool. Use the questions to evaluate the playground. Does the playground measure up? Is there a need for change? Where? What will that change involve?

Then, prepare a plan for bringing your current playground into conformity. Transfer the theoretical plan questions and check sheets into a format that will be easy to use at various predetermined intervals in the future. This will enable professionals to maintain the playground in compliance with reasonable standards for participants' rights and negligence

A professional is encouraged to share the risk management plan with the agency's insurance company and retained attorney. Many agencies will employ a playground consulting firm to examine the plan and the environment for adequacy in risk planning.

Should an injured party file a law suit, the agency and the professional will use the results of their risk management planning as evidence of the standard of care on the playground. Reports of the adequacy of the plan provided by external consultants will be used by attorneys in preparing a defense and could be introduced into a court of law.

In summary, professionals are encouraged to know civil rights law, particularly ADA, and standards for negligence and to recognize that plans need to be made to assure the civil rights of participants and to establish a standard of care. Rights and standard of care are implemented and practiced at all times. Evidence, in writing, of assurance of rights and standard of care is prepared and used if the playground professional is challenged.

References

Bauer, Eugene G., & Ronald Pinegar. (1987). *The primer for playground safety*. Grinnell, IA: Ashley Scott & Assoc.

Black, Henry Campbell. (1979). *Black's law dictionary*. 5th ed. St. Paul, MN: West Publishing Company.

Bruya, L.D., & Langendorfer, S.J. (Eds.). (1988). *Where our children play: Elementary school playground equipment*. Reston, VA: AAHPERD.

Clement, Annie. (1988). *Law in sport and physical activity*. Carmel, ID: Brown and Benchmark.

Dunn, John M. (Ed.). (1991). PL 99-457, challenges and opportunities for physical education. *Journal of Physical Education, Recreation and Dance, 62*(6), 33-48.

Keeton, W. Page, Dobbs, Dan B., Keeton, Robert E., & Owens, David G. (1984). *Prosser and Keeton on torts* (5th ed.). St. Paul, MN: West Publishing Company.

Moore, Robin C. (1987). *Play for all*. Berkeley, CA: MIG Communications.

Perritt, Henry H., Jr. (1990). *Americans with Disabilities Act handbook*. New York: Wiley Law Publication.

Thompson, Donna & Bowers, Louis (Eds.). (1989). *Where our children play: Community park playground equipment*. Reston, VA: AAHPERD.

Thompson, Donna. (1991). Safe playground surfaces: What should be used under playground equipment? *Journal of Physical Education, Recreation and Dance, 62*(9), 74-75.

United States Consumer Product Safety Commission. (1991). *A handbook for public playground safety*. Washington, DC: U.S. Government Printing Office.

Wortham, S.C. & Frost, J.L. (Eds.). (1990). *Playgrounds for young children: National survey and perspectives*. Reston, VA: AAHPERD.

Zimroth, Peter L. (1991). *The Americans with Disabilities Act, planning for compliance*. New York: Practicing Law Institute.

Camping for Individuals with Disabilities: Standards and Guidelines

Susan F. McConnell

Camping programs have been supplementing therapeutic and educational programs since long before legislative mandates. However, many individuals with disabilities have been unable to fully participate in all aspects of camping activities due to existence of barriers. Passage of the Americans with Disabilities Act (P.L. 101-336) of 1990, the most comprehensive piece of disability civil rights legislation enacted since the Civil Rights Act of 1964, affects the majority of camps and camping areas in the United States. Individuals with disabilities can no longer be excluded from camping experiences. Neither attitudinal, nor informational, nor physical barriers to full participation experiences may continue to exist.

Everyone has different talents and abilities; each person has the right to access and choice of recreational opportunities that best suit their needs. The Easter Seal Society of Wisconsin, in its staff guides for Camp Waubeek and Pioneer Camp, has defined the basic rights for individuals with disabilities.

> This camp-oriented summary of the ADA should not be construed as legal opinion; legal counsel should be consulted for full interpretation of the law.

In recreation and leisure, individuals with disabilities have the right to:

- Experience positive recreation and leisure pursuits.
- Experience the normal range of individual experiences.
- Experience independence and self-reliance.
- Experience normal peer relationships.
- Have atypical needs met.
- Have it recognized that their needs may be as great as, if not greater than, the nondisabled individual when opportunities have been denied previously.

In camping and in outdoor and environmental recreation, individuals with disabilities have the right to:

- Appreciate their relationship to the natural world.
- Participate in a camping, outdoor, or environmental recreation experience.
- Achieve growth and developmental potentials through quality camping experiences.
- Participate in family camping experiences.

In camping and in outdoor and environmental recreation, individuals with disabilities have the need to:

- Experience growth and development that may have been previously denied to the disabled.
- Experience independence from regular caregivers.
- Experience successful activities.
- Recognize their relationship to the natural world.
- Experience relationships extending beyond the camping experience.
- Receive direct leisure education instruction.
- Learn carryover recreation and leisure skills and activities.
- Build self-confidence.
- Have proper preparation to allow for the most beneficial experience possible. (Easter Seal Society of Wisconsin)

Each individual with a disability has basic rights to access and participate in camping, outdoor, leisure, and recreational activities, and these rights have been aided by passage of the Americans with Disabilities Act of 1990 (ADA). This Act mandates that facilities and programs be made available to individuals with disabilities. This means that private and public sector providers of camping and outdoor education/leisure opportunities must make their facilities and services accessible to *all* persons, including individuals with disabilities. This chapter explores the rights of individuals, the responsibilities of providers, and practical factors for implementation of accessible programs in the areas of day camps, resident camps, outdoor recreation areas, parks and forests, and commercial camping facilities.

Camping and the ADA

Camping provides opportunities to bring individuals with disabilities into the mainstream. In the informal, nonthreatening atmosphere of camping there are opportunities for interaction between individuals with disabilities and their nondisabled peers, fostering friendships and experiences that might not happen in other settings.

In the 1970s and 1980s many camps were slow to integrate individuals with disabilities. A variety of factors were involved in this negative situation, including:

- Lack of knowledge and experience in working with individuals with disabilities.
- Fear of the unknown.
- High costs of removing architectural and environmental barriers.
- Need for higher staff to camper ratios.
- Staff discomfort with integrating individuals with disabilities into existing programs.
- Lack of staff training in techniques to ensure all campers receive quality experiences.
- Attitudinal barriers of camp staff, parents, campers, and the general public.
- Fear of how to deal with possible problems.

Camps and camp programs are now required to be accessible to all persons. Camps will be unable to discriminate against employing qualified individuals with a disability. The ADA provides comprehensive civil rights protection to individuals with disabilities in the areas of employment, public accommodations, state and local government services, and telecommunications. Title I—Employment, and Title III—Public Accommodations and Services Operated by Private Entities (including transportation) have particular implications for camps.

Title I—Employment

Employment applies to all camps: private, agency, religious, for-profit and nonprofit. Camps having 25 or more full-time employees who work 20 or more weeks out of the year, or camps owned by an agency or religious group employing 25 or more full-time employees must have met Title I by July 26, 1992. Some states have additional and more stringent regulations. For example, the New Mexico Human Rights Act contains provisions similar to those of the ADA and applies to employers of four or more employees. Check each state for additional legislation.

Exceptions include:

- Corporations owned entirely by the U.S. government.

- An Indian Tribe.
- A private club (exempt from taxation under section 501(c) of the IRS code of 1986. A private club (camp) cannot be organized for the purpose of being excluded from the law.

Smaller camps and businesses are given a longer time for compliance. Camps having 15 to 24 full-time employees have until July 26, 1994 to comply. Agency and religious camps owned, controlled by, or having trustees elected from parent bodies are not excluded from the less than 15 employees rule if there are more than 15 employees in the parent body.

When individuals with disabilities are employed by camps and are involved in camp program planning, camp programs can become much more meaningful for campers and staff. Who better to provide challenges for campers with disabilities than staff with disabilities? Camp staff with disabilities can serve as role models for campers in addition to providing ideas of what works and what does not in camp programming.

Individuals with disabilities who are protected against discrimination are people considered to have one of the following:

- A physical or mental impairment substantially limiting one or more life activities.
- A record of such an impairment.
- Being regarded as having such an impairment.

No business/corporation may discriminate against a qualified individual with a disability who satisfies skills, experience, education, and other job-related requirements and who, with or without reasonable accommodations, is able to perform essential functions of the job an individual either wants or holds. This means that absolutely no discrimination against an individual with a disability in regard to job applications and procedures, hiring, advancement, discharge, compensation, job training, and other terms, conditions, and privileges of employment will be tolerated by this mandate.

No camp can:

- Use administrative criteria to discriminate on the basis of disability.
- Deny services to persons known to have association with individuals with disabilities.

- Apply eligibility criteria that will screen out individuals with disabilities, unless criteria are necessary to provide the service.
- Contract with an employment agency or another agency providing training or fringe benefits that discriminates against an individual with a disability.
- Discriminate against a person who refuses to participate in discriminating behavior or who has participated in a proceeding or investigation under the ADA.

An employer may not ask an applicant about the nature or severity of disability. However, an employer may ask about the applicant's ability to perform job-related functions and may ask for a demonstration. Medical examinations after employment are allowed if all employees must have the same examination. A test for illegal drugs is not considered a medical exam.

An applicant or employee who is an illegal drug user is not covered under the ADA. However, an individual who has undergone a supervised rehabilitation program or who has been successfully rehabilitated and is no longer abusing drugs may be considered a "qualified individual with a disability." An employer may prohibit illegal use of drugs at the workplace and/or require employees not be under the influence of alcohol or illegally used drugs in the workplace.

Auxiliary aids may be requested by camp employees with disabilities.

An employee with a visual impairment might request:
- adaptive computer software.
- electronic visual aids.
- braille devices.
- magnifiers.
- audio recordings.
- signs in braille.
- curbs on trails.
- qualified readers.
- large print materials.

An employee with a hearing impairment might request:
- telephone headset amplifiers.
- TDD equipment (telecommunications for the deaf/text telephone).
- telephones compatible for hearing aids.
- lights on emergency alarms.

- closed caption decoders.
- assistive listening devices.
- a qualified interpreter.
- video text displays.

An employee with mobility impairment might request:
- ramps.
- grab bars in toilet and shower facilities.
- wider aisles.
- larger parking areas accessible to each worksite.

An employee with dexterity limitations might request:
- raised/lowered furniture.
- gooseneck telephone headsets.
- mechanical page turners.

Camps must be prepared to make reasonable accommodations to known limitations of an otherwise qualified individual with a disability who is an applicant or employee, unless undue hardship on the operation of the camp can be demonstrated. Reasonable accommodation means making present facilities accessible, restructuring job descriptions, purchasing modified equipment, providing interpreters, or similar accommodations. Undue hardship exists if modifications would change the nature of services provided or cause undue financial burden. Readily achievable means it is easy to accomplish without much difficulty or expense. Effective dates for the above are: July 26, 1992 for employers with 25 or more employees; July 26, 1994 for employers with 15 to 25 employees.

Employers may not discriminate against qualified individuals with disabilities and must reasonably accommodate them. Enforcement policies and procedures exist. Persons claiming to be discriminated by an employer, potential employer, or business may file a complaint with the Equal Employment Opportunity Commission (EEOC) within 180 days of the alleged violation. After the complaint is filed:

- The EEOC must notify the person charged with the violation within 10 days of the date of filed charges.
- The EEOC will investigate and if violations are found make recommended resolutions.
- If the violation is not resolved, the person who was discriminated against may sue in Federal District Court or the Attorney General may choose to sue the violator.

Camps and their owner/administrative body need to look at hiring practices and policies to ensure the nondiscrimination intent of the ADA is being met.

Using phrases such as able-bodied, duties as delegated, and driver's license required will not help a camp director select the right person for a camp position and will not give the potential employees reasonable expectations of what they may expect on the job.

The ADA mandates no discrimination against persons who are able to fulfill the essential functions of the job, with or without reasonable accommodation. This means camp directors or camp administrators must define in writing all essential functions of the job, for each position within the camp or outdoor setting.

The American Camping Association in *Camping Magazine* (March/April, 1992) has recommended that camp management staff conduct a self-evaluation of services offered, programs, activities, staff training, and facilities to determine where barriers exist and what needs to be done to overcome these barriers. Camp management should include individuals with disabilities to help brainstorm ideas on how to accommodate staff with disabilities in their program.

Title III—Public Accommodations and Services Operated by Private Entities

No camp or camping area may deny individuals with disabilities opportunities to participate in or benefit from its services. No camp or camping area may fail to provide individuals with disabilities opportunities equal to opportunities, services, and facilities provided to nondisabled individuals.

Day and Resident Camps

Camps may provide separate facilities and services for individuals with disabilities, if separate facilities and services are necessary to provide opportunities for individuals with disabilities. However, it must be stated in brochures that separate programs for individuals with disabilities are provided. ADA mandates that individuals with disabilities cannot be denied access to integrated programs even if separate programs are provided.

Factors used to determine whether removal of barriers is within what is reasonable accommodation include:

- Nature and cost of effort required to remove barriers.
- Overall financial resources of camp facilities in question.
- Effect of barrier removal on expense, resources, and camp operation.
- Overall financial resources of the camp's parent body; overall size of the workforce.
- Number, type, and location of other facilities owned by parent body.

All camps are included in this mandate except camps with religious sponsorship while serving their specific religious group. Some religious camps may have to voluntarily comply with Title III in order to continue operating with their present clientele. Public schools, Scout groups, Easter Seal, and other like groups that fall under Title III will not be able to rent or lease a camp, even a religious camp, not meeting ADA Title III provisions. The burden of proof will be up to owner/operators renting or leasing accessible facilities.

In order to compete in the marketplace camps will need to comply with the intent of the law. Camps receiving USDA surplus commodities, special milk, summer feeding program, or camper assistance funds program are under obligation to be accessible under Section 504 of the Rehabilitation Act (National Camp Executives Group. 1992. p. 4).

This does not mean every area and every program has to be barrier free. If the barrier cannot be removed with reasonable accommodation because of expense, or because it would change the camping experience, alternative accommodations must be created to meet the intent of the law. Newly developed areas and buildings must be accessible.

Camps will need to be creative in their approach to all campers. By making camps barrier free, camp programs can be accessible to all. The ADA requires that within a camping program, opportunities must be the same for individuals with disabilities and nondisabled alike. With good programming it is possible with some modifications in implementation to have camping experiences be similar for campers with disabilities and the nondisabled. A nondisabled camper needs to gain understanding and acceptance of the camper with a disability. With good role models and program accessibility this can happen.

Plans need to be developed as soon as possible to enable all camps to come into compliance. Requirements will be based on size of camp, resources available, length of time camp has been in operation, clientele served, and staff training.

Not every building has to be made accessible; however, some of the sleeping cabins, bathing/toileting areas, the health care facilities, dining lodge, and some program areas must be barrier free. Paths to these areas must also be accessible for individuals with disabilities. This does not mean camps must spend large amounts of money to accomplish this; however, thought must be given to integrating campers with disabilities into all regular camp activities and into peer appropriate living units.

Implications of the ADA for building and property changes is based on terrain and local conditions. Camp facilities need to be designed for the highest level of accessibility practical for any given site. With increasing numbers of individuals with disabilities participating in camp activities it just makes good sense to design accessible buildings and facilities. When doing a site and property management plan or update, decisions should be based on the degree to which a site can be developed, and/or modified, for use by all people.

Camping Areas

The National Park Service and U.S. Forest Service are developing state-of-the-art design guides to assist camp owners and operators in dealing with how to rid facilities of barriers. Accessibility varies from easy accessibility to most difficult (primitive camping), enabling all levels of participation. The Special Programs and Populations Branch of the National Park Service has made significant efforts to make our National Parks accessible for all.

Family camping for a family with a person with a disability is now possible. More and more campgrounds have physically accessible campsites. Families with a disabled person can now enjoy a wide range of family camping experiences, from the desert to the wilderness to the seashore. Several resources are available on accessible camping areas:

- *National Parks: Camping Guide* for a list of parks with accessible sites. The guide is available from local Government Printing offices or from the Superintendent of Documents, Government Printing Office, Washington, DC, 20402-9325. (Price is $4.00.)
- *Design Guide for Accessible Outdoor Recreation,* U.S. Department of Agriculture and U.S. Department of the Interior, Government Printing Office.
- *Easy Access to National Parks: The Sierra Club Guide for People with Disabilities* (1992), Wendy Roth and Michael Tompane. The Sierra Club, San Francisco, CA. $16.00.
- *Easy Access National Parks,* VHS Video, available from National Park Foundation - Video, 1101 17th St., NW, Suite 1102, Washington, DC 20036. $19.00 plus $3.00 shipping and handling.

Facilities must be designed so they can be approached, entered, and used by all persons with disabilities. Physically accessible sites must provide a place to park, accessible paths of travel, minimum doorway openings of 32 inches, and accessible restrooms. Services and information offered to nondisabled visitors must be accessible to them. Information accessibility is just as important as physical accessibility. Program accessibility is just as important as bathroom accessibility. Newly constructed or renovated facilities must comply with Code 41 of Federal Regulations (CRF) 101-19.6 of the Uniform Federal Accessibility Standards.

The National Park Service and the U.S. Forest Service have developed *Design Guide for Accessible Outdoor Recreation* (in press). It is a state-of-the-art resource on accessibility. It includes an Accessibility Evaluation Survey, a checklist to use when evaluating a site for accessibility. There is also specific, detailed technical data, including information on technical capabilities of elements and materials for accessible outdoor recreation facilities.

Four levels of accessibility are addressed:

- Easy, usable without assistance.
- Moderate, usable with some assistance.
- Difficult, semi-primitive.

- Most difficult, primitive, offers a higher level of risk and challenging experience.

A resource for manufacturers of accessible outdoor drinking fountains, toilets, pumps, firegrates, water spigots, etc. is also planned. For more information, contact:

USDA Forest Service; Auditors Bldg.
Attn: Access Coordinator, Recreation
2011 14th Street, SW at Independence Ave., SW
Washington, DC 20250
202-205-1129 or 202-205-1706

Levels of accessibility for camps and outdoor recreation trails are influenced by physical characteristics of the site: slope of trail, surface materials used to make the trail, and the amount and type of safety features needed. Persons with mobility limitations as well as persons with visual impairments may have problems with accessibility, but not necessarily the same problems. All individuals with disabilities will need to be addressed when redesigning old or designing new facilities.

An accessible facility must offer persons with disabilities an opportunity to have experiences similar to those offered nondisabled individuals. When designing or modifying facilities, the use of the universal design is the preferred approach since it considers all persons, not just the average. Universal design means considering all degrees of sensory awareness, all types of mobility, and all levels of physical and intellectual functioning when planning and designing facilities. Structural changes to buildings have until January 26, 1995 to be in compliance.

A campground operator who rents park trailers, tents, or recreational vehicles may have an obligation under the ADA to make a number of rental units accessible for use by campers with disabilities. In addition, the campground operator may have to provide accessible vehicles if removal of existing barriers is not readily achievable (NCOA, 1991 p. 5).

Camp Accreditation

The American Camping Association (ACA) serves as a consultant and advisor to state and federal agencies related to day and resident camping. In addition it serves in an advisory capacity in the areas of outdoor education and recreation to colleges and universities.

Since 1935 the American Camping Association (ACA) has developed standards of compliance for camps voluntarily seeking accreditation. The purpose of the ACA Camp Standards Program is to assist camp directors and camp owners in providing quality camping experiences for campers and staff and to assist the general public in selecting camps meeting industry-accepted and government-recognized standards. When a camp is accredited, it means the owners/operators have voluntarily invited an outside team of ACA trained visitors to verify compliance in all applicable areas of camp operation including site, administrative practices (including transportation, emergency procedures, food service), personnel, program, health care, and some specialized activities (American Camping Association, 1990, p. 4).

Camps must also meet local, state, and federal regulations pertaining to camp operation. When those regulations require a level of performance different from the ACA standard, the higher requirement must be met by the camp. In addition, agency camps may also have standards or guidelines recommended by their national organization.

In order to be an accredited American Camping Association camp, the camp must be in full compliance with all applicable mandatory standards and score at least 80% in each applicable section of the standards pertaining to the camp's program, site, and operation. Visitations must occur when the camp is in full operation. Accredited camps are visited at least once every three years to verify compliance to ACA standards. It must be noted, however, that while ACA standards focus on health and safety, there is no guarantee that a camper attending an accredited camp is totally free from harm.

Resources

For camp standards —

Standards for Day and Resident Camps
American Camping Association
5000 State Road 67 North
Martinsville, IN 46151-7902

For complaints —

Complaints should be in writing, signed by person making complaint or an authorized representative. Include the name, address, and description of the alleged discriminatory action. Send to:

Coordination and Review Section
Civil Rights Division
U.S. Department of Justice
P.O. Box 66118
Washington, DC 20035-6118

Complaints may also be sent to the appropriate agencies designated for enforcement of Title II:

- Department of Education for complaints regarding education systems and institutions other than health-related schools and libraries.
- Department of Interior for complaints regarding lands and natural resources, including parks and recreation, water and waste management, environmental protection agency, historic and cultural preservation, and museums.
- Department of Labor for complaints regarding labor and the work force.

For specific information —

For information about ADA requirements affecting telecommunications contact:

Federal Communications Commission
1919 M St., NW
Washington, DC 20554
202-632-7260 (Voice)
202-632-6999 (TDD)

For information about ADA requirements affecting transportation contact:

Department of Transportation
400 Seventh St., SW
Washington, DC 20590
202-366-9305 (Voice)
202-755-7687 (TDD)

Selected References

American Camping Association. (1990). *Standards for day and resident camps.* Martinsville, IN: American Camping Association.

Bedini, L.A., Bialeschki, D., and Henderson, K. (1992). Americans with disabilities: Implications for camp programming. *Camping Journal,* 64. 53-58.

Easter Seal Society of Wisconsin (n.d.) *Pioneer camp staff guide.* Madison, WI: Easter Seal.

Hedley, E. (1979). *Boating for the handicapped: Guidelines for the physically disabled.* Albertson, NY: Human Resource Center.

National Campground Owners Association Education Foundation. (1990). *Americans with disabilities act: A campground operator's guide to compliance.* Reston, VA: NCOA Education Foundation.

National Camp Executives Group. (1992). *Camp director's primer.* Monticello, NY: Markel Rhulen Underwriter's & Brokers.

Plourde, R. (n.d.) *Access Information Bulletin.* Paralyzed Veterans of America. Recreation. Washington, DC: Paralyzed Veterans of America.

Scanlin, M.M. (1992). Better camping for all. *Camping Journal,* 64. 28-34.

United States Department of Agriculture, United States Department of Interior. (Interim draft, 1990). *Design guide for accessible outdoor recreation.* Washington, DC: Government Printing Office.

United States Department of Justice. (7/26/91). *Federal Register,* part III. 28 CRF Part 36.

ACA Camp Standards
Relating to Campers with Disabilities

The American Camping Association, a private, nonprofit educational organization, is the only nongovernmental group to set standards, procedures, and guidelines for observing practices of member camps. The standards below (*Standards for Day and Resident Camps*, 1990) are those that pertain to the ADA requirements and the operation of accredited ACA camps. Standards are presented in the form of questions, followed by an interpretation and demonstration of compliance.

A-13 — Are sleeping, dining, toilet, and program facilities available to persons with disabilities, or is the camp implementing a plan to come into compliance with the Americans with Disabilities Act?

Interpretation: The intent of this standard is for the camp to address facility accessibility issues as defined by the Americans with Disabilities Act of 1990. The law does not require all facilities or program areas be accessible, or that all changes be made at once. The ADA law does not require camps to make changes that would fundamentally alter the nature of the camp program. It does require the camp to make "readily achievable" accommodations that do not cause an "undue burden."

It may not be possible to make all areas of camp accessible. However, participation in the normal activities of camp living and activity groups should be fostered and barriers removed or accommodations provided to permit full participation whenever possible. "Available" means persons have both access and opportunity.

Compliance Demonstration: Director explanation of plans established and/or accommodations provided for persons with disabilities.

A-19 — Are toilets adequate in number based on the following ratios:
1. One seat for every 10 females.
2. One seat for every 10 males, and
3. If more than 10% of camp population has restricted mobility—
   a. One seat for every 8 females, and
   b. One seat for every 8 males?

Interpretation: Seats to be used in computing toilet ratios are those available to general camp population and not those in private residences or restricted areas. Up to one third of the seats for males may be substituted with urinals.

Compliance Demonstration: Visitor observation of randomly selected toilet areas; director/staff explanation of ratios available. (ACA, p. 24).

A-21 — (does not apply if a primitive camp) Do bathing/showering facilities provide:
A. Adequate numbers—
1. All camps — one showerhead or bathtub for each 15 persons in camp, or
2. Camps specializing in serving persons with restricted mobility — one showerhead or bath tub for each 10 persons in camp?

Interpretation: "Primitive camp" refers to camps whose program is based on a philosophy centered on nonfacility, utility-oriented principles. Generally, such camps have few permanent structures or facilities.

Bathing facilities to be used in computing ratios are those available to the general camp population and not those in private residences or restricted areas.

For persons with restricted mobility, aids such as chairs on casters, stools, footrests, nonslip surfaces, and flexible shower heads attached to hoses may provide increased independence. Aids should be provided according to the needs of persons being served.

Compliance Demonstration: Visitor observation of randomly selected showering/bathing areas and devices for those with restricted mobility (if applicable); director explanation of ratios acceptable. (ACA, p. 25).

A-22 — (does not apply if structures are not used for sleeping quarters) Do permanent sleeping quarters provide the following:
1. Cross ventilation,
2. At least six feet between heads of sleepers,
3. At least 30 inches between sides of beds, and
4. Adequate space to provide freedom of move ment, especially for those using wheelchairs or walkers?

Interpretation: "Permanent sleeping quarters" refer to structures, platform tents, covered wagons, etc. that are constructed in a fixed location and are used as primary residences for staff and campers. Temporary shelters such as tents for overnight camping and back-packing would not fall under this classification.

Beds separated by less than 30 inches but having a fixed partition between them that preclude sneezing or coughing on others is acceptable to meet the standard.

All persons need adequate space for ease of movement and to facilitate safe exit in an emergency. State regulations range from 30 to 50 square feet of floor space required per person. Such regulations should be considered when designing, constructing, or using buildings.

Persons with restricted mobility need additional space and the arrangements should consider functional space taken by wheelchairs and other devices themselves.

For persons with restricted mobility, the norm established by ANSI is 50 square feet per person using a walker and 60 square feet per person using a wheelchair.

Compliance Demonstration: Visitor observation of randomly selected sleeping quarters throughout camp. (ACA, p. 25-26).

C-1 — Does the on-site director have the following qualifications:
A. A bachelor's degree or an ACA Camp Director Certification?
B. At least two prior seasons of administrative or supervisory experience in an organized camp?
C. If camp primarily serves campers with special needs, 24 weeks of experience working with special populations?
D. Attended workshop, institute, seminar or course related to camp management, camper or staff development, and/or environmental education within the past three years?
E. At least 25 years of age?

Compliance Demonstration: Director explanation of qualifications. (ACA, p. 49).

C-2 — (does not apply if camp does not primarily serve campers with special needs) Do 20% of the camp administrative personnel and program personnel with staff supervisory responsibilities have a bachelor's degree in an area relevant to the clientele served or at least 24 weeks of experience working with the special populations being served?

Interpretation: Serving campers with special needs requires skills and experience beyond what is required for other camp operations. The intent of this standard is to provide a minimum level of specialized training and experience at the administrative and staff supervisory levels.
Compliance Demonstration: Director explanation of camp's percentage. (ACA, p. 49).

C-5 — (does not apply if camp does not serve campers with physical, medical or behavioral needs who require additional staff support to participate in camp, e.g. physically or mentally disabled, emotionally disturbed, etc.) Are procedures being implemented that require:
A. Ratios of staff and counselor-support personnel that meet or exceed the following?

Camper Age	Staff	Resident Campers	Day Campers
4-5 years	1	5	6
6-8 years	1	6	8
9-14 years	1	8	10
15-18 years	1	10	12
19 & over	1	20	20

B. At least 80% of the ratios established in part A be met with personnel 18 years of age or older?

Interpretation: Camps may not categorically refuse to serve persons who require additional staff support (see current DNA). However, all camps may not serve persons requiring these levels of supervision, for various reasons. Therefore, the standard cannot be scored consistently as currently worded. Since the ADA specifies additional staff assistance as a "readily achievable" accommodation to make for persons with special needs, the ratios in the chart should be used as a guideline in determining appropriate personnel support when such persons are served. (ACA 1992, Addendum).

C-9 — Are procedures in practice for informing all staff of specific needs of campers for whom they are responsible?

Interpretation: The intent is that all appropriate staff be informed of medical, physical, or other needs or restrictions of campers under their supervision, cabin or in program activities. This may include information on diet, allergies, medications, rest requirements, and activity restrictions; recognition and care of potential medical problems such as choking, seizures, and hypoglycemia; care and handling of campers with wheelchairs, prosthetic, and orthopedic devices; and any other specialized needs or limitations of individual campers.

Compliance Demonstration: Director/staff description of training; visitor observation of general camper/staff interactions. (ACA, 1990, p. 54).

E-4 — Is written evidence available which shows camp health manager is qualified as follows:

Day Camps

1. Is a licensed physician or registered nurse, or has access by phone to a licensed physician or registered nurse with whom prior written arrangements have been made in writing to provide consultation and/or other medical support to the camp; or

2. If the camp serves primarily persons with special medical needs — Is a licensed physician or registered nurse; or

3. If a nonmedical religious camp — Is an individual meeting qualifications specified in writing by the religious program?

Resident Camps

1. Is a licensed physician or registered nurse, or is in consultation with a licensed physician or registered nurse who is on the campsite daily, or

2. If camp primarily serves persons with special needs — Is a licensed physician or registered nurse who is on duty at all times, or

3. If a nonmedical religious camp — Is an individual meeting qualifications specified in writing by the religious program?

Interpretation: For Day Camps: In part 1, access by phone should be to a specific doctor, nurse, or clinic who is familiar with the camp's health care needs. Access to a 911 emergency phone system does not qualify as access to specific medical personnel who are providing on-going consultation to oversee camp health.

For Resident Camps: In part 1, the daily consultation may include such things as checking current health concerns or recent treatments and reviewing the medical log and/or accident reports.

"On the campsite daily" means there is time each day when a person so licensed is on the property to consult with the health care staff, review actions taken, and provide further guidance in implementing the camp's Health Care Plan.

Nurses and doctors who are not licensed to practice in the camp's locale are qualified to meet this standard only if they are temporarily licensed or recognized by the state in which the camp is located. Camp directors are advised to check the applicability of malpractice insurance to non-U.S. trained or licensed personnel.

For camps primarily serving persons with special needs, provision must be made for similarly qualified substitutes when the physician or RN must be away from camp for more than 12 hours in a resident camp or more than 1 day in a day camp. For periods less than this, a licensed practical nurse or a graduate nurse may be used.

Compliance Demonstration: Visitor observation of appropriate licenses, authorizations, or written arrangements where appropriate; director description of arrangements/scheduling. (ACA, 1990, p.79-80).

E-16 — (does not apply if camp does not primarily serve persons with special needs) To meet the special medical needs of participants, are the following available:

A. Sufficient medical staff to meet the needs of participants equivalent to minimums established in the Appendix; or if ratios are not addressed in the Appendix, health care staff as approved in writing by a licensed physician?

B. A system for evaluating the camp's ability to meet participants' special medical needs prior to enrollment?

C. Information about camp's philosophy and health management practices that is shared with parents/participants prior to enrollment so they can identify the camp's approach to medical concerns?

Interpretation: "Special medical needs" include all disabling conditions which require special medical or health attention or care while the participant is in camp including chronic conditions such as insulin-dependent diabetes, or epilepsy; illness such as cancer; physically disabling conditions such as spina bifida; etc. (ACA, 1990 p. 86).

F-13 — (does not apply when persons in wheelchairs are not near bodies of water, natural or constructed) Is there a procedure in practice requiring that seatbelts or ties be removed from persons who are in wheelchairs while in watercraft or near bodies of water?

Interpretation: "Near bodies of water" includes all locations from which there is a possibility of the chair rolling into the water.

Compliance Demonstration: Visitor observation of activities when possible; staff description of procedure utilized with persons in wheelchairs. (ACA, 1990, p. 98).

American Camping Association, Inc., 1990. *Standards for Day and Resident Camps.* Martinsville, IN: American Camping Association, Inc. Reproduced by permission.

Suggestions for Making Camp Buildings and Facilities Accessible

A camp director or administrator needs to take a long, hard look at existing property and facilities. A camp evaluation is necessary. A list follows containing suggested items to consider. It gives camp administrators a place to start in determining what accessibility changes are necessary and what will be achievable. Not every building must be accessible, but buildings providing important services for all campers, such as dining lodge, health center, shower facilities, and some program areas, must be accessible. Any new construction project must be accessible.

Ecological barriers include the physical obstacles present in any natural environment. If it is physically impossible to remove the barrier then an alternative method of access must be created. It will take careful thinking and planning to remove ecological and architectural barriers.

Building and Site Accommodation Checklist — Suggested Items

Information listed below was adapted from information obtained from USDA (1990).

Unit Living Accommodations/ General Buildings

Outside Area

- ramps to buildings
- handrails inside and outside building
- 32 inch wide doorways (all doorways including toilet stalls)
- flush thresholds
- doors opening to 90 degrees
- easy to open doors—needing less than 8 pounds pressure
- 5 foot level clearance in direction of door swing
- U-shaped door handles/lever handles
- indoor and outdoor tables without benches
- standing cooking grills in addition to fire circles

Parking Area

- one 8 foot wide parking area with 5 foot access aisle
- total spaces

Parking Spaces	Accessible Spaces
1 to 25	1
26 to 50	2
51 to 75	3

- parking areas 96" wide with 5' aisle and universal disabled parking sign
- dropoff parking zone

Inside Area

- hallways 51" wide to allow for wheelchair turning
- hallways free of obstacles and clutter
- nonslip flooring
- telephone, operational parts no more than 48" from floor
- room names/numbers/information in braille
- water fountains should have height of 36" from floor, use a lever operational with one hand

Restrooms

- accessible toilet and area with space for transfers—51 inches min (60" x 60")
- toilet seats 17" to 19" from floor (no spring seats)
- sinks and counter 29" above floor
- sink handles easy to use, levers are best
- soap dispensers, towels no more than 34" from floor
- width of doorway: 32 inches
- outward door swing to 90 degrees
- soap dispenser, towel dispenser/blower, mirror: 40 inches from floor
- toilet stall: 3' x 4' x 8' with 32" or wider doorway with grab bars on either side of toilet, and/or in back

Shower Area

- accessible shower area with space for transfer, 60" x 60"
- shower chair
- flexible showerhead

- nonslip floor
- water thermostatically controlled by temperature regulating valves
- changing table/bench
- mirrors/dispensers no higher than 40 inches from floor

Dining Lodges (see unit living accommodations for specifics)

- ramp to building
- parking area
- toilet facilities on 1st floor
- seating arranged to accommodate wheelchairs
- signage

Paths/Ramps

At the time of writing, no official standard for trails existed. One accessible route should be provided from public street/road to each accessible building. All buildings should be connected by paths having the following characteristics:

- must be level (no stairs)
- width: 36 inches
- passing space for 2 wheelchairs of 5 feet every 200 feet if trail is less than 5 feet
- rest areas (benches every 200 to 300 feet/ shelter desirable)
- edging on outside of trail/path to aid visually impaired using a cane
- surface material may be concrete, pavers (brick or tile) set on concrete base, asphalt, crushed s tone, wood decking, or soil cement (soil, sand, mixed with cement and steam rolled).
- ramps, should have incline of 1 foot rise in 12 inches/5% grade, have hard, nonslip surface that will not rot, have minimum of one handrail 32" high extending 1 foot beyond top and bottom of ramp.
- signs should have raised letters, include braille/ tactile (words/maps) presentation, have con trasting colors and clear headspace—80 inches (USDA, 1990).

Camp Program Areas

Arts and Crafts

- accessible tables with space for wheelchairs
- accessible sinks and faucets
- accessible equipment and supplies

Aquatics

General Waterfront Area
- accessible toilet
- ramp and level dock area
- accessible path to area
- pathway from parking to beach
- firm stable path (asphalt, concrete, wood plank 4 to 5' wide
- handrails 30-34" high (may restrict maintenance vehicles)
- signage

Pathway from beach to water
- stabilized sand or wood plan—less impact on beach (stabilized sand with hardened clay must be reconstructed each summer)
- handrails may obstruct view (use with discretion)

Access to water
- handrails 30-34" high
- wheelchairs available and designed to go into water
- large rubber mat directly on the sand can improve access to water (less support to swimmers, less subject to water erosion)
- signage
- means of transfer from wheelchair to dock/ water with grab bar

Swimming
- access to the area
- level docks/ramps
- transfer to the water (sand is unstable)

Boating
- access to the area
- transfer area
- shore transfer (sloped area/hard nonslip surface; 8.3% grade or 1:12)
- fixed dock transfer (dock no higher than 18 inches above water)
- floating dock transfer (dock no higher than 18 inches above water/floating docks may be more unstable)
- access to the water's edge
- safety equipment

Swimming Pool
- accessible parking area
- accessible firm paths
- ramp or extra wide steps as options for patrons for water entry
- slip-resistant walkway areas throughout pool area
- slip-resistant stairs and 3' wide ramps (8.3% grade or 1:12) with handrails on both sides

- 18" block of stairs with 6" high risers with 18" tread
- use color and texture to indicate edges/high risk areas, mark increase in water depth
- signage (information and safety)
- use of color for float markers/lane lines/dividing areas

Bathhouse area
- wheelchair available designed to go into water for ramp and shower use
- 36 inches between bench and lockers
- nonslip floor area
- use of color and texture to indicate pool and ramp edges
- large benches for seated and reclining dressing

Campcraft

- accessible campsite
- accessible grill that rotates, 30" from ground
- accessible fireplace grate should be 18 to 24" from ground
- hard surface around grill
- accessible table with tops extending 19" from legs at a height of 29" from ground level with 3' clearance on both sides
- accessible water source with faucet height 36 to 40" from ground level, placed on hard surface that does not get soft when wet. Use lever controls on faucet, drain grate openings should be less than 1/2 inch
- accessible drinking fountains with lever controls, located 34 to 36"

Ceremonial Fires and Campfires

- accessible area with backed benches and room for wheelchairs
- accessible fireplace grate 18" to 24" from ground level
- hard surfaced area

Equestrian Activities

- access to location of horses
- transfer areas onto and off horses
- access to the facilities to facilitate care of horses
- accessible facilities to water hydrants and corral gates
- mounting platform to enable disabled riders to mount and dismount at stirrup level
- 24 inch high platform, 5' x 5'
- ramp with 1 1/2" diameter handrail 30" x 34" high

Fishing

- access to the area
- access to water's edge (hard, nonslip; sand is unstable)
- shade
- space for gear
- dock with curb (2", 4" when no guard rail present)
- guard railings (42" high for standing and 32" for seated areas and children)
- benches
- 8 foot minimum width of dock

Nature

- accessible paths and trails
- exhibit space should be barrier free
- exhibits at comfortable viewing level
- hard ground surface area, level, and slip resistant
- signage should have large type, panel colors designed to reduce glare, tent information and graphics should be easy to understand and read
- trail guides available on tape or in braille

Sports Fields

- accessible area
- accessible paths and trails to area
- playing surface should be level
- accessible toilets
- areas of shade
- accessible drinking fountains
- accessible toilet facilities
- accessible equipment storage areas
- accessible equipment available
- signage as needed

Guidelines, Regulations, and Standards for Play Equipment and Surfaces

Donna Thompson

This article discusses available guidelines, regulations, and standards for play areas, play equipment, and surfacing under equipment, with special attention to providing facilities accessible for children with disabilities. Standards exist in order to provide an appropriate environment for safe play; they indicate a concern for care for individuals. Governing bodies making standards include the United States, state, and local governments and professional associations. Those who do not follow standards may provide a hazardous environment and may be sued. Teachers, administrators, and recreators need to know existing standards, which can carry the force of law. Use standards in order to force producers to make better equipment, and purchase only from producers complying with standards and guidelines.

Play Areas and Equipment

In November 1991, the United States Consumer Product Safety Commission (USCPSC) issued its *Handbook for Public Playground Safety*. Although it is only a guideline, suggesting minimums, it is considered "the standard" against which to measure information about playground equipment and surfacing. It was written for consumers with the understanding more technical aspects for manufacturers would be written in the American Society for Testing and Materials (ASTM) Standard. For equipment, it gives information about layout, design, materials, construction, access of platforms, major types, use

zones, and surfacing. Information is based on injuries children have sustained and hazards to avoid in order to prevent recurrence of those types of injuries. Appendices include a suggested general maintenance checklist, entrapment requirements and test methods, characteristics of surfacing materials, and descriptions of loose-fill surfacing materials. This handbook can be ordered from the U.S. Consumer Product Safety Commission, Washington, DC 20207, or by calling 1-800-638-2772.

The handbook does not give any information in relation to playground equipment about interpretation of the Americans with Disabilities Act of 1990. It indicates that "specific federal requirements for accessibility to playgrounds by the disabled are expected to be published," but as of this writing, that has not been done.

Home Playground Standards

The American Society for Testing and Materials (ASTM) sponsors the development and publishing of standards of various types. The latest version of the Standard Consumer Safety Performance Specification for Home Playground Equipment, F 1148-91, was completed in 1991. It is a technical standard of requirements for home playground equipment for children from ages 2 through 10. It is not intended to apply to equipment to be used in places of public assembly such as schools, nurseries, day care centers, and parks. While it does give information about playground equipment for home use, it does not refer to equipment that could be adapted for children with disabilities.

Those interested in influencing accessibility changes might like to serve on that committee in the future. The committee is composed of any interested parties, including manufacturers, and must have 50% of its constituents from the consumer, general interest area so decisions have input balanced with those from the manufacturing industry. That requirement is true for all ASTM standards in terms of composition of subcommittees. The Home Playground standard is in the process of being revised and a new edition will probably be available in 1993. For information, contact Teri Hendy, Chair, Home Playground Standard, ASTM, 1916 Race St., Philadelphia, PA 19106.

Public Use Playground Standard

The American Society for Testing and Materials F15.29 Subcommittee to Develop a Public Use Playground Equipment Standard has been in existence since May 1988. It is in the process of developing a technical standard for public use playground equipment, which is being developed in conjunction with the U.S. Consumer Product Safety Commission's *Handbook for Public Playground Safety*, published in 1991. It is nearing completion of its work and the subcommittee hopes to have a standard published during 1993. One section under consideration deals with accessibility for children with disabilities. The subcommittee has met with representatives from the U.S. Park Service and has been asked to interpret the Americans with Disabilities Act in regard to playground equipment. If that section is included in the standard, it will probably be the document used to interpret ADA in regards to playground equipment for children with disabilities. For information, contact Fran Wallach, Chair, Public Use Playground Standard, ASTM, 1916 Race St., Philadelphia, PA 19106.

Child Care Programs

The American Academy of Pediatrics and the American Public Health Association combined to make National Health and Safety Performance Standards: Guidelines for Out-of-Home Child Care Pro-

grams (1992). They are described in *Caring for Our Children*, which cites some spacial dimensions, describes some placement suggestions and heights of fences, and provides general information about maintenance. There is a very brief section about "Playground and Outdoor Areas of the Facility" and about "Surfacing of Playground and Outdoor Areas," but there are no references about accommodating children with disabilities.

State Laws

The state of California is the only state that has passed a law governing purchase of playground equipment. As of 1991, California requires that all playground equipment purchased for public playgrounds conform to USCPSC Guidelines contained in the *Handbook for Public Playground Safety* (1991) and that all types of play activity in new and redone play areas be accessible to individuals with disabilities. In the absence of references on one's own state, readers could conclude that, under ADA, the minimal standards for all children would apply to children with disabilities.

Those considering purchasing equipment are encouraged to refer to their own state regulations regarding accessibility. The state of Iowa, for example, is in the process of developing a law to regulate purchasing of playground equipment in relation to the USCPSC *Handbook for Public Playground Safety* (1991), the ASTM Standards, and the Americans with Disabilities Act.

A handbook, *Analysis of State Regulations for Playgrounds and Their Supervision*, by Fran Wallach and Susan Edelstein, with results of a survey about all regulations about playgrounds and elementary schools, parks ,and childcare centers is now available from the National Recreation and Parks Association, 2775 S. Quincy St., Arlington, VA 22206, 703-820-4940.

Surfacing

The U.S. Consumer Product Safety Commission's *Handbook for Public Playground Safety* (1991) contains a section on surfacing as related to injuries resulting from falls from equipment. The section does not address surfacing as it relates to mobility. The American Society for Testing and Materials Public Use Playground Standard is expected to address the issue of mobility.

The ASTM standard now describes critical height of equipment in proportion to an impact of peak deceleration of no more than 200 Gs and a Head Injury Criteria (HIC) of no more than 1000 when tested in accordance with technical procedures described in ASTM F1292. These are two different measurements used to determine that an injury may be life threatening and a way to measure the impact a head may have in landing on a surface. The procedure was used in connection with several loose fill materials and the results of those tests are noted. When purchasing surfaces, it is important that the surface maker be able to produce test results using F1292 and F355 test methods, with information to indicate how high equipment can be in proportion to the depth of the surface. Anyone considering refurbishing an established play area should use materials from producers who can show the same kinds of results from testing using the F1292 and F355 methodology.

Further, the Americans with Disabilities Act indicates that new play facilities must be accessible for wheelchairs. One should check with the producer to be certain a surface does provide mobility for a wheelchair.

The American Society for Testing and Materials (ASTM) has created a standard to systematically evaluate surfacing materials for use on playgrounds. Impact attenuation deals with the force with which an object, such as a head, hits the surface and the ability of the surface to absorb the hit. It is the intent of the standards to present information for manufacturers to measure the impact of an object and thus the thickness of material needed to prevent a child from being injured seriously, such as a receiving a concussion, or dying. The standard is to be used by manufacturers of materials to measure and then by potential buyers to compare results of measurements in order to determine which materials to purchase. A user or adult child-care giver should ask for test results of the product and be sure tests were done in accordance with F1292, which is the standard Specification for Impact Attenuation of Surface Systems Under and Around Playground Equipment. If results are compli-

cated, users should ask for the information to be interpreted in a manner similar to the chart in the USCPSC *Handbook* (1991, p.21).

There are only four places in the United States equipped to perform this test: Northwest Labs, Pennsylvania State University, Michigan State University, and University of Indiana. The cost may be as much as $3,000, but it is still important that tests be done in order to verify depth of material needed in relation to height of equipment used. An appropriate depth of material may prevent a concussion, which is basically what the 200 G level and the HIC test of 1000 means, in lay terms. Other injuries are also less likely to occur. Both loose fill and unitary materials should be tested.

There is a standard test method for shock-absorbing properties of playing surface systems and materials which should be used in the F1292 procedure noted above. Buyers should look for the use of this method in the report given in regard to shock-absorbing qualities of the surface one is considering.

Although these two standards are very technical in nature, and the typical lay person is not expected to understand the test method, buyers should look to see that those tests were performed on products they are considering. Sellers are likely to refer to the fact that they use test results of other manufacturers, or just gloss over the fact and say their product meets all ASTM Standards, but that is impossible since all standards ASTM produces do not apply to playground surfaces.

Wheelchair Accessibility

There are some loose fill products that are wheelchair accessible. Mats or unifill materials that are used under and around playground equipment are not the only appropriate products. Be sure to ask about mats that are used with playground equipment. They are not the same as gymnastic mats. Request verification and names of buyers to check out the seller's assertion that the product will allow wheelchair mobility. However, individuals in wheelchairs do not need to be able to get to the entire area. Surfacing must allow users access to a representative amount of play equipment, not necessarily to all. Thus, all surfacing does not need to be wheelchair accessible.

If the site was built after January 1991, wheelchairs do need to be able to get to the area and surfacing must allow them to move to get into position to get onto some equipment. Areas built prior to 1991 are required to be accessible; however, allowances may be made for situations where undue financial burden exists and/or where making an area accessible would significantly alter the experiences made accessible.

Playground Surface Companies

When considering surfacing materials, ask the company to provide you with testing results that have used ASTM F1292 and F355 methods and, as a result, can provide you with the ratio of the depth of the product to the height of the equipment that you intend to provide.

Inclusion of company names does not imply endorsement of any product by the author or publisher.

Appollo Safety Surfaces, 3386 Durahart St., Riverside, CA 92507

Astroturf Industries, 801 Kenner St., Dalton, GA 30720

Baker Rubber, Inc., Box 2438-T, South Bend, IN 46680, 219-291-5101

Breakfall, 759 N. Milwaukee St., Milwaukee, WI 53202, 414-273-7828

California Products Corp., 169 Waverly St., PO Box 569, Cambridge, MA 02139

Cam-Turf, Safeplay, 9th Floor, Republic Bank Tower, 15301 Dallas Parkway, Dallas, TX 75248, 214-851-7033

Carlisle Tire & Rubber Co., P.O. Box 99, Carlisle, PA 17013

Child Safe Safety Surface, 55 Lamar St., W. Babylon, NY 11704, 516-491-5577

Evergreen Landscape Nursery, Wood Mulch, Dale L. Peterson, Mgr., 4000 Blairs Ferry Rd., NE, Cedar Rapids, IA 52402, 319-395-0144

The Fibar Systems, 838 West Street, Harrison, NY 10528, 800-FIBAR-21

The Mat Factory, Inc., 760 W. 16th St., Suite E, Costa Mesa, CA 92627, 714-645-0966; 800-628-7626

Midwest Elastomers Inc., P.O. Box 412, Wapakoneta, OH 45895

Mitchell Rubber Plastics, 23-31 94th St., East Elmhurst, NY 11369

Mitchell Rubber Plastics, 491 Wilson Way, City of Industry, CA 91724

Monarch Rubber Co., 3500 Pulaski Highway, Baltimore, MD 21224

Playfield Industries, Security Blanket Playground Surfacing Division, Box 1564, Williamsville, NY 14231-1564, 800-685-play

Play Safe Surfaces, Inc., 240 West Bristol Lane, Orange, CA 92665, 714-974-0783

Pyco Regeneration Systems, Inc., Clark Maritime Centre Bldg., 5100 Utica Pike, Jeffersonville, IN 47130

Rochester Chemical & Mat Company RCM, Box 604, Anoka, MN 55303, 612-421-0129; 800-328-9203

RoseBar, Shredded Rubber Mulch, Box 106, Vinton, IA 52349, 319-472-5271

Safe Site, 5995 Harrison Ave., Cincinnati, OH 45248

Safety Surfaces, 937 Kirkland Ave., Kirkland, WA 98033

Safety Turf, Inc., Box 820, Oaks, PA 19456, 215-666-9186

Sparton Enterprises, Shredded Rubber Mulch, 3717 Clark Mill Road, Barberton, OH 44203-1099, 216-745-6088

Sportec International, Inc., 1491 Sheridan Drive, Kenmore, NY 14217

Tire Turf Systems Inc., Box 186, Harlan, IN 46743

TuffTurf, Landscape Structures, 601 7th St., Delano, MN 55328, 800-328-0035

Uniroyal Chemical Co., Spencer St., Bldg. 112, Naugatuck, CT 06770

Uniroyal, Inc., 312 N. Hill St., Mishawaka, IN 46544

Supply & Equipment Companies

When asking for catalogs, ask for three kinds: preschool or child-care settings; elementary school or park settings; and children with disabilities. Each is geared to a different audience and covers different items.

Inclusion of company names does not imply endorsement of any product by the author or publisher. Some of the names were made available verbally from the National School Supply and Equipment Association, 8300 Colesville Road #250, Silver Spring, MD 20910, (301) 495-0240. NSSEA makes lists of supply and equipment companies available to its members.

Accessibility Design Information Center, University of Nevada, Reno, NV 89557, 702-784-1499

American Playtime Systems, Inc., Playlinks, 7 Knight Hill Court, Melville, NY 11747-3909, 800-231-PLAY

Big Toys, 7717 New Market St., Olympia, WA 98501, 800-426-9788, 206-943-6374

B.C.I. Burke Co., PO Box 549, Fond Du Lac, WI 54935, 414-921-9220

Children's Playgrounds, Inc., 55 Whitney, Holliston, MA 07466-6159, 800-333-1588

Columbia Cascade Timber Co., 1975 South West Fifth St., Portland, OR 97201, 503-223-1157

GameTime, Inc., PO Box 121, Ft. Payne, AL 35967, 205-845-5610

Gerber Leisure Products, Inc., Box 5613, Madison, WI 53705, 800-236-7758

Hags Play, USA, 6458 Fiesta Dr., Columbus, OH 43235

Iron Mountain Forge, PO Box 897, Farmington, MO 63640, 800-325-8828, 314-756-4591

Kompan, Inc., RR 2 Box 249, Marathon, NY 13803-9802, 800-553-2446

Landscape Structures, Inc., Rt. 2, Box 26, Delano, MN 55328, 800-328-0035, 612-972-3391

Miracle Recreation, Hiway 60 at Bridal Lane, Box 420, Monett, MO 65708, 417-235-6917

Parity, Inc., Box 3593, Oak Park, IL 60303

Playworld Systems, PO Box 227, New Berlin, PA 17855, 717-966-1015, 800-233-8404

PCA Industries, 5642 Natural Bridge, St. Louis, MO 63120, 314-961-5110

Quality Industries, Inc., Hillsdale Industrial Park, PO Box 765, Hillsdale, MI 49242-0765, 517-439-1591

See-Saw-Snake, Box 14, Boulder, CO 80306

Topper Industries, Battleground, WA

Video — *Inspecting Playgrounds for Hazards*, The Information Exchange, Box 1528, Fair Oaks, CA 95628, 800-443-8373

References

American Public Health Association & American Academy of Pediatrics (1992). *Caring for our children: National health and safety performance standards: Guidelines for out-of-home child care programs.* Washington, DC & Elk Grove Village, IL.

California State Law: Senate Bill No. 2773, Chapter 1163, September 20, 1990, effective, January, 1992.

Moore, R.C., S.M. Goltsman, & D.S. Iacafano (Eds.). (1987). *Play for all guidelines: Planning, design and management of outdoor play settings for all children.* Berkeley, CA: MIG Publications.

Public Law 101-336. Americans with Disabilities Act. 26 July, 1990. *Federal Register.*

Public Law 101-336. 104 Stat. 327 (July 26, 1990).

Standard Consumer Safety Performance Specification for Home Playground Equipment, F 1148-91. (1991). Philadelphia, PA: American Society for Testing and Materials.

Standard Specification for Impact Attentuation of Surface Systems Under and Around Playground Equipment, F 1292-91. (1991). Philadelphia, PA: American Society for Testing and Materials.

Standard Test Method for Shock-Absorbing Properties of Playing Surface Systems and Materials, F 366-86. (1991). Philadelphia, PA: American Society for Testing and Materials.

Critical Issues: Risk Management, Informed Consent, and Participant Safety

Julian U. Stein

Physical educators, coaches, recreation leaders, and others responsible for physical activity programs have long been concerned with safety of participants in their programs. However, adequate and appropriate standards of care for the past are neither adequate nor appropriate today. Legal requirements and court precedents now place much greater responsibilities upon prudent professionals—and volunteers—than at any previous time.

Too many recreation leaders—whether in regular or special programs—do not take all steps necessary and mandated to acquaint program participants with potential dangers in activities. Such procedures—especially those related to risk management, informed consent, and participant safety—are required of individuals responsible for any type of physical, recreation, leisure, sport, and activity programs, not just activities considered to be high risk such as ropes and challenge courses, white water rafting, mountain climbing, or sky diving.

Seattle Case judgments (Adams, 1982, 1985) have identified rather clearly definitive responsibilities of leaders—administrators, teachers, coaches. Even though the Seattle Case involved a high school football player who became a paraplegic through an injury suffered in practice, court judgments were worded in ways that apply equally to interscholastic sport programs, school-centered physical education, and community based recreation programs, regardless of sponsors—community recreation departments, youth sport clubs, or community organizations such as YM/YWCAs.

Although at this point we are not aware of any court cases involving private agencies or pay for play programs in which Seattle Case principles have been specifically applied, every prudent and professional leader, regardless of sponsoring organization or agency, should be aware of and apply these principles and procedures in every activity in their programs.

As increasing numbers of individuals with disabilities enter and participate actively in virtually any and every physical, recreational, leisure, and sport activity, care and concern for risk management programs, informed consent, and safe participation must be given high priority. Judgments of the Seattle Case have no limitations to specific populations—they have generic implications and applications to all populations, including individuals with disabilities.

Therefore readers should apply Seattle Case principles and processes to their programs involving participants with disabilities, whether individuals are integrated into regular programs or are in self-contained, segregated, adapted settings. Specific interpretations and applications of Seattle Case principles and procedures for individuals with disabilities have been incorporated throughout this document to assist readers in developing and implementing sound risk management activities in their own programs.

This article is an expansion of *Injury Precaution Sheets: You Can't Afford to Be Without Them* (Julian U. Stein), which was published in *The Virginia Journal* (journal of Virginia Association for Health, Physical Education, Recreation, and Dance), April 1991, and later reprinted with permission in *The Indiana Journal for Health, Physical Education, Recreation, and Dance* (journal of the Indiana Association for Health, Physical Education, Recreation, and Dance), Spring 1991.

Implications and Applications of the Seattle Case

Judgments of the Seattle Case applicable to programs and activities sponsored by groups such as those presented above include the mandate to:

- Spell out to program participants in very specific terms the dangers involved in physical, recreational, leisure, and sport activities, regardless of level or sponsor.
- Require each staff member to be aware of all latest safety techniques relevant to every activity taught or coached.
- Check each staff member's knowledge and proof of adequate participant conditioning, lead-ups, and progressions for every activity taught or coached.
- Review with each staff member proper techniques in skill teaching and performances in every activity.
- Place an emphasis on injuries, including those of a catastrophic nature, that are possible if proper technique is not used in the activity. (Adams and Bayless, 1982)

In practical terms, what does each of these factors mean? Exactly what is expected of teachers, coaches, and program leaders—including those responsible for programs and activities involving participants with disabilities—to be in compliance with judgments of the Seattle Case? Specifically, those in leadership positions, including administrators, in physical activity and sport programs must:

- Develop and implement a detailed risk management program that includes contact information at every activity site about each program participant; information about medications, allergies, seizures, specific disabilities, and contraindicated medications for use in case of an accident or other emergency involving program participants.
- Have a readily available emergency action plan at every activity site that includes information about how to contact parents/guardians/care takers/specified neighbors, ambulance, rescue squad, police, fire department, and other emergency medical personnel.
- Develop, distribute, and discuss injury precaution sheets for each activity, tailored according to unique and specific characteristics and factors of the activity (see later section in which injury precaution sheets are discussed in detail).
- Be sure each staff member—paid professional or volunteer—is aware of latest safety techniques (including regular and special equipment, application of rules, skill execution, and appropriate and neces- sary safety accommodations and precautions for participants with disabilities) for each activity taught or coached. This requires acceptance of dual responsibilities, those of program leaders and administrators.

Program leaders must have basic preparation incorporating knowledge and promoting necessary attitudes about risk management procedures and injury precautions for each participant in every activity. This basic preparation must be supplemented regularly and on ongoing bases through reading appropriate professional journals, attending workshops and clinics, and keeping safety of program participants as a primary priority.

Program administrators must make it possible for program leaders to obtain professional journals and materials and to attend conferences, workshops, clinics, and other inservice activities, including those dealing with safety involving individuals with disabilities. Administrators should also be sensitive to these needs and include, in both regular and special inservice activities, programs and sessions dealing with all aspects of safe participation.

- Order subscriptions to journals and newsletters such as *From the Gym to the Jury* (The Center for Sports Law and Risk Management, 8080 North Central Expressway, Suite 400, Dallas, TX 75206); *Exercise Standards and Malpractice Report* and *The Sports, Parks and Recreation Law Reporter* (both from Professional Reports Corporation, 4571 Stephen Circle, NW, Canton, OH 44718); *Fitness Management* (Leisure Publications, Inc., 3923 West 6th Street, Los Angeles, CA 90020), which includes Law Notes in each of its monthly issues. Administrators responsible for physical, recreational, leisure, and sport programs should obtain such periodicals and develop ways to ensure program leaders read and use these as well as other appropriate resources regularly.
- Be sure program participants are provided with appropriate and necessary basics for each activity—conditioning, warm-up, lead-ups, progressions, and cool-down. Detailed daily lesson or practice plans with appropriate notes regarding actual implementation, revisions, and individual accomplishments and accommodations are basic to planning and conducting programs that are safe for all participants. Accommodations for participants with disabilities must be considered in this process.
- Be sure program leaders remain current of changes in rules and skill execution techniques—including those related to activities and sports for individuals with different disabilities—so all program participants are assured of the latest and safest techniques related to each activity.
- Make safety an ongoing consideration in every activity, including discussions with program participants at the beginning and during the activity

and injury precaution sheets shared with program participants and, in the case of minors, their parents or guardians. Injury precaution sheets must be understandable for all participants and available in accessible formats (large print, audiotape, braille, captioned slides, and/or videotapes) for participants with various disabilities.

Legal Responsibilities of Leaders and Administrators

Standard of Care

Teachers, coaches, and leaders must offer students, athletes, and program participants an appropriate standard of care to protect them from harm. Such a standard of care is expected to be that which any reasonable and prudent qualified professional with comparable background, training, and experience would apply under similar circumstances. Generally, each state determines and defines background, training, and experience of qualified personnel, including bases for licensure, certification, endorsement, or registration. Teaching skill, discretion, and knowledge that qualified members of the profession in good standing normally possess in similar situations are examples of factors considered in establishing a standard of care for given situations (Dauer & Pangrazi, 1989).

Professional training, background, experience, and specialization are additional considerations. "Qualified" for program leaders with participants with disabilities in their programs would, at a minimum, signify basic knowledge of and about program participants with disabilities and their conditions. The more severe the conditions of program participants, the greater the expectation for higher levels of knowledge and competence. In addition, professional personnel in therapeutic or clinical programs would be held to quite a different standard of care from personnel in community based recreation programs. Standard of care comparisons are made with those in comparable programs and activities, and with similar background, training, and experience.

An individual with specific training, background, and experience in coaching would be held to a higher standard of care than a volunteer coach. However, this does not give volunteer coaches carte blanche to approach their duties and responsibilities in ways that exceed their training, background, and experience. For example, an individual with no knowledge or experience in tumbling and gymnastics would have difficulty in justifying teaching or coaching front or back flips, especially in court after a program participant has been injured. An individual with no first aid or CPR training would be asking for trouble to use a tourniquet to control bleeding or administer CPR.

Program administrators are asking for legal difficulties if they assign program leaders to conduct and supervise activities for which they do not have sufficient training, background, and experience. If confronted with such a situation, programs leaders should object, stating they do not have appropriate background and competence to teach or coach the activity. If the program administrator continues to insist, then the program leader has no alternative but to write a letter of objection to the assignment with appropriate reasons and rationale. This letter should be placed in the program leader's permanent personnel file as documentation to his/her objection to the assignment. This, in most cases, shifts responsibility from the program leader to the program administrator, in case of a negligence charge.

Foreseeability

A trained professional is expected to be able to foresee potentially dangerous and harmful situations. Was it possible for the teacher to predict and anticipate the danger of the harmful act or situation and take appropriate measures to prevent it from occurring (Dauer & Pangrazi, 1989)? For example, an individual with Down syndrome openly exhibits fear and says she does not want to attempt a basic vault. When the program leader insists that she try, an ensuing injury would, indeed, have been foreseeable.

Equipment (permitting children to use playground apparatus that is faulty, does not have appropriate or sufficient ground cover, or has protruding rusty nails or bolts), facilities (leaving unattended rope courses so they can be used by any passerby), teaching progressions (demanding hand springs before students have been successful with various types of forward rolls), and supervision (leaving students on their own in locker and shower rooms or unsupervised in activities) all relate to foreseeability. Nothing can be left to chance. If an injured individual can prove a teacher, leader, or coach should have foreseen danger involved in an activity, that individual could be found negligent for failing to act in ways of a reasonable and prudent professional.

Foreseeability can, indeed, be a double-edged sword, especially when serving program participants with disabilities. On the one hand, the individual with a disability has the right to participate. On the other hand, the program leader must be concerned with safety of all participants, including those with disabilities. Individuals—disabled or not—should be kept out of activities, or permitted to participate only at more basic levels, when personal safety is threatened in specific activities.

Disability in no way negates foreseeability. While a program leader is justified in prohibiting an individual with a disability from taking part in a given activity, such decisions should be based on safety considerations, not generically made on the basis of disability. Decisions to prohibit an individual with disabilities from trying or taking part in an activity should be based on the individual's lack of skill, proficiency, or fitness, in the same ways similar decisions would be made for any program participant, disabled or not. Appropriate uses and applications of various accommodations must be considered.

Basic Factors of Negligence

Four basic factors must *all* be present if an individual is to be judged negligent (Appenzeller, 1978):

- Duty or responsibility to an individual. Program leaders by nature of their positions—paid professional, volunteer, or administrator—have a duty to everyone in their programs. A program leader having little or no training in working with persons with disabilities is not absolved of duty or responsibility to program participants with disabilities.
- Breach of duty from failure to fulfill one's responsibilities to program participants. Such a breach can be in any of a number of ways—failure to provide appropriate instruction, inadequate supervision, failure to warn of inherent dangers in the activity itself (see section on injury precaution sheets, and/ or inappropriate or no risk management plan. Program participants and their parents or guardians have the right to expect qualified leadership in all activities, including necessary training to deal with disabilities and their impacts on specific activities.

In legal terms, breaches can be misfeasance— following proper procedures, but not according to the required standard of conduct, usually subpar performance of an act that might have been lawfully

done (e.g., not spotting properly during a tumbling or gymnastic routine); malfeasance—doing something improperly by committing an act that is unlawful and wrongful (e.g., paddling a student for misbehavior when such acts are contrary to local or state laws); or nonfeasance—doing nothing (lack of action) in carrying out a duty, an act of omission in which a leader knew proper procedures but failed to follow them (Dauer & Pangrazi, 1989).

- Injury to the individual. Even if a duty has been breached, if there is no injury, there is no basis for negligence. If a duty has been breached and there is no injury, program leadership can consider itself lucky, and should learn and benefit from this luck.
- Proximate cause between breach of duty and injury. This is usually the crux of a court case, establishing a cause and effect relationship between breach of duty and injury.

Recent court cases in general, and the Seattle Case in particular, have done nothing to change these four factors or relationships among them in negligence cases. However, specific aspects of one's duties and responsibilities to program participants have been much more clearly identified and defined, especially as related to such areas as risk management and informed consent. These same factors have implications for and applications to program participants with disabilities, as no distinctions are made as to whether or not individuals are disabled.

Defenses Against Negligence

Various factors have been valid defenses against negligence, including (adapted from Appenzeller, 1978):

- Assumption of risk in which a program participant—or parents or guardians of a participant when the participant is under 18 years of age—accepts risk of potential injury. Parents or guardians of individuals with low mental functions can be expected to assume risk for participation of their children or wards. An individual with only one eye, kidney, or lung who wants to participate in a contact sport, such as football or wrestling, cannot be denied opportunity to participate on the basis of having only one of paired parts. While the sponsoring agency has responsibility to alert the individual to potential catastrophic dangers if the remaining part is lost, the decision to participate or not is that of the individual. "Pursuant to long-standing legal principles, some children under specific ages (7 to 14) are either conclusively or rebuttably presumed to be incapable of assuming the risks associated with their participation in various sports or activities or in being self-negligent" (Herbert, November 1991, p. 26).

- Contributory negligence in which a program participant is guilty of negligent behavior so negligence of the defendant is negated and charges dropped. Only two states still have contributory negligence provisions; comparative negligence (see next section) is the standard throughout the other 48 states. Presence of a disability, even in high risk activities, is not in and of itself considered a contributing factor in case of injury. Key phrase is negligent behavior, as basis for contributory negligence.
- Comparative negligence in which a program participant is guilty of negligent behavior so compensation is prorated according to proportion of plaintiff and defendant degrees of negligence. When this is the situation, either judge or jury, depending upon how judgment is to be determined, assesses degrees of plaintiff and defendant negligence. Reviews of cases in a number of states did not reveal any apparent formula for determining degrees of responsibility of plaintiff and defendant. However, in some states if percentage of plaintiff negligence exceeds that of the defendant, no monetary recovery can be obtained by the plaintiff.
- An act of God in which some unforeseen and uncontrollable act, such as lightning, gusts of wind, or a cloudburst, creates a situation which results in injury to a participant. Key words here are unforeseen and uncontrollable. An act may be uncontrollable, but foreseeable! For example, during a softball game lightning and thunder are seen and heard at a distance. A prudent umpire would suspend the game at this point, not wait until lightning and thunder get closer. "The act of God defense can be used only in those cases in which injury would still have occurred had reasonable and prudent action been taken" (Dauer & Pangrazi, 1989, p. 143).

Historically, the best defenses against negligence have been those showing absence of one or more of the four factors that must be present for negligence to be adjudged. Totally fulfilling *all* duties of one's position and responsibilities to *each* program participant is probably the best defense against negligence, including such factors as proper instruction, appropriate supervision, adequate planning, and necessary background, training, and experience for working with program participants having disabilities. Such duties and responsibilities cannot be attained adequately today without special attention to risk management and informed consent.

In many ways the Seattle Case (Adams, 1985; Adams & Bayless, 1982) has greatly reduced, if not

rendered moot, many traditional defenses against negligence. Age of program participant, for example, is an important consideration if assumption of risk is to be a valid defense against negligence; an individual must be old enough and sufficiently mature (mental age might be an appropriate guideline for program participants with cognitive disabilities) to know what risks are being assumed.

Activities of a required instructional physical education program, participation in involuntary intramural and interscholastic programs, as well as mandatory recreation activities, regardless of sponsor or setting, do not lend themselves to an assumption of risk defense. Without an appropriate and adequate informed consent and risk management program, assumption of risk becomes far less effective as a defense against negligence.

The Law and a Potpourri of Considerations

Releases

Laws relating to warning statements and participant releases are changing, vary from state to state, and are undergoing rapid development in some states. Basic principles regarding releases apply equally to individuals whether or not they possess disabilities. However, releases cannot be required of program participants with disabilities if they are not required of participants without disabilities.

Recent court decisions have presented diametrically opposite decisions regarding validity and value of release forms.

- Use of releases by a weight-loss facility was upheld by a court decision. "The use of contractual release documents can greatly limit a facility's exposure to certain kind of suits in some jurisdictions where the use of these documents is recognized and if they are properly worded, read, and executed according to requirements of law. In the long run, the proper development and utilization of these forms can go a long way to reduce risk of claim and suit" (Herbert, May 1991, p. 23).
- The Virginia Supreme Court ruled, "The law in Virginia has been settled that an agreement entered into prior to any injury . . . is void because it violates public policy" (the first court ruling relating releases and public policy found anywhere in the United

States). This ruling has been generally interpreted throughout Virginia to mean injury waiver forms are probably not worth the paper on which they are printed. Negligence or personal injury cannot be contracted away (Zambito, 1992).

- In a recent case, a husband's release did not prevent his wife and children from suing over injuries suffered by the husband/father in a race-car accident (Herbert, June 1992). The court held, "The right is her separate and personal right arising from the damages she sustains as a result of the tort feasor's conduct. The right of the wife to maintain an action for loss of consortium occasioned by her husband's injury is a cause which belongs to her and which does not belong to her husband."

Regardless of legal status, releases provide important positive public relations and information about activities to program participants, their parents, guardians, and families. Based on recent judgments, it would be wise to plan accordingly and develop release forms after consultation with legal counsel to ensure the forms and procedures will be effective and prevent needless claims and suits (Herbert, June 1992).

Individuals signing such releases must be sufficiently mature (chronological or mental age) to understand both the release and risks being assumed. In no way can recent developments be interpreted as legalizing negligent behavior on the part of a teacher, coach, or program leader. From this standpoint, little, if anything, has changed. In addition, applications of the Americans with Disabilities Act (1990) make it necessary for release forms to be presented in ways individuals with disabilities can understand and use (large print, audio cassette, braille, signed interpretation).

Inherently Dangerous Activities

Various activities, such as graded exercise testing procedures that are virtually routine in many health clubs, exercise programs, and spas, can be deemed *inherently dangerous* under certain circumstances. The basic issue is whether staff members have a duty to warn program participants of risks involved in undergoing such procedures as a stress EKG, especially when the individual has potential complicating conditions such as diabetes, obesity, or previous history of heart disease (Herbert, June 1991).

A basic question arises that must be closely followed in the future through the courts. Will stress EKG procedures be considered inherently dangerous under all circumstances? While there may be attempts to have these procedures declared to be inherently dangerous in particular cases, this would be contrary to the vast available scientific literature in favor of such procedures under appropriate conditions. However, health and fitness facilities dealing with individuals having serious medical histories, or where there are contraindications for such procedures, should refer such individuals to appropriate medical practitioners before proceeding (Herbert, June 1991).

A recent Colorado case emphasizes risks arising from water-based activities in a club setting (Herbert, May 1992). The wife of a club member who died of brain surgery associated with oxygen deprivation from being partially submerged in a whirlpool charged the facility "in failing to warn of the risks and hazards associated with the use of a whirlpool." Even though the verdict in this particular case was for the club, such facilities have certain professional obligations to program participants, including "duty to inform, warn, supervise, and periodically monitor those involved in hot tub, spa, and whirlpool use. Anything less may well expose facilities to substantial claim and suit." It should be noted that standards related to spa use have been developed and are available from the U.S. Consumer Product Safety Commission and the American College of Sports Medicine.

What is an inherently dangerous activity? This is a difficult question to answer. Some activities are in and of themselves inherently dangerous. Other activities may be inherently dangerous for some individuals, with or without disabilities. Still other activities may be inherently dangerous without properly trained and qualified leadership.

Even improperly assembled equipment can be considered inherently dangerous. A New York jury awarded an injured plaintiff $500,000 because of an improperly assembled exercise bicycle that caused her injuries (Herbert, February 1992). This case clearly points out the need "to adopt an exercise equipment assembly and inspection policy—one that ensures proper assembly in accordance with the manufacturer's requirements, an inspection after assembly, and a testing mechanism prior to placing the equipment into use. Anything less may well be deemed negligent." Such a procedure, complete with adequate records as to assembly, inspection, and testing, should be part of regular risk management programs.

To provide safe, sound, and sane programs for every participant, with or without disabilities, one should approach each activity as if it is, in fact, inherently dangerous for all participants. Introducing and implementing an appropriate injury precaution sheet program is an important factor in this process.

Exercise Testing Procedures

A recent statement issued by the American Heart Association and American College of Cardiology defines "the minimum education, training, experience and cognitive and technical skills necessary to the competent performance of exercise testing . . ." (Herbert, April 1991, p. 42). This statement is certain to affect the standard of care for exercise testing procedures.

The position statement calls for physician supervision of such procedures, even for what some exercise and sport science professionals might consider to be fitness assessment purposes. The statement recognizes that in certain situations and under given circumstances exercise testing can be safely performed by trained personnel working under the direct supervision of a physician. Those who may perform such procedures under physician supervision are limited to nurses, exercise physiologists, physical therapists, or medical technicians. The physician must be in the immediate vicinity and available for emergency response.

An important question regarding standard of care for graded exercise procedures is raised for health clubs and fitness facilities—who may perform such procedures? This statement could well be used to attack performance of such procedures by nonspecified personnel. Facilities should review this new statement with legal counsel and compare its effect upon existing state law regarding unauthorized practice of medicine.

Another recent publication, *Personal Trainer Manual, The Resource for Fitness Instruction* (American Council on Exercise) provides information as to "trainer duties in screening and evaluation of clients; development and design of safe exercise activities for clients; and provision of safe instruction and adequate supervision" (Herbert, March 1992, p. 27). This publication provides information and materials on programming for healthy adults, as well as for special populations. "While this work seems to have

been written for resource and self-teaching purposes (to prepare some readers for ACE's certification examinations for personal trainers), it clearly will have implications to the standard of care owed by this professional population to their clients."

Additional standards and statements recently released by the American Heart Association (*Special Report: Exercise Standards, A Statement for Health Professionals from the American Heart Association*) and the American College of Sports Medicine (*Guidelines for Exercise Testing and Prescription*) "provide the professional framework within which exercise testing and prescription must be carried out by health and fitness facilities" (Herbert, April 1992, p. 16). Facilities "should engage in recommended screening procedures. Those which offer more than intake screening services should ensure their procedures and policies for testing, prescription and supervision for various populations adhere to these authoritative expressions."

Unsupervised Children

Recent developments make it incumbent on health centers, exercise clubs, spas, and other activity facilities to develop appropriate policies and procedures for protecting bystanders—especially children—and individuals who use weight training/lifting equipment. Even though a facility appropriately provides activities for participants of all ages, certain activities must be judged to be inappropriate for young children, and only appropriate for older children when properly supervised. Muscular endurance training for children should only be permitted when conducted by well-qualified adults. Therefore, the standard of care expected requires that children be excluded from some facility areas and that proper supervision is provided for older children (Herbert, November 1991).

The United States Consumer Product Safety Commission issued an alert to keep children away from exercise bikes. Warnings should include points such as:

- Keep children away from exercise bikes.
- Never use a bike without a chain guard.
- Store the bike where children cannot get to it when not in use (Herbert, December 1990).

While this discussion has focused on weight training/lifting equipment and exercise bikes, all facilities with various exercise devices and machinery must ensure that children—especially toddlers and prepubescent youth—are kept away from such equipment, unless properly supervised at all times. "Failure to consider such policies and precedents, and to adapt them for facility use, would seem to be below the applicable standard of care" (Herbert, November 1991, p. 26).

Specific considerations may have to be given program participants having mental ages of children, but with adult chronological ages. Such individuals should not be considered children, for they possess physical qualities and have had various experiences quite different from children with the same chronological and mental ages. While difficult, if not impossible, to generalize about such individuals, treat each as an individual, do not insult their chronological ages and intelligence (remember many of these individuals have a great deal of street smarts), and if erring, err in the direction of chronological, rather than mental, age.

Off-Site Activities

Sponsors who take program participants to other indoor facilities or outdoor spaces are responsible for an appropriate standard of care during activities away from their own facilities. Foreseeability of potential problems, as exercised by a reasonably prudent professional with comparable background, training, and experience, is a key factor involved in protecting program participants, whether activities are at or away from the basic program site (Herbert, August 1991).

These responsibilities include facility sponsored or recommended activities on jogging trails, activity paths and certain off-site activities that may be encouraged—such as jogging on streets or roads or going to various eating establishments. Duty also includes safe accessibility for program participants to and from the home facility. In areas where there is likelihood of attack, precautions need to be instituted so as to avoid such potential situations. When such opportunities are offered, facilities must consider safety of program participants insofar as the area of activity is concerned. Off-site facilities must be accessible in every way for individuals with disabilities.

"Facilities would be well advised to ensure that their recommendation of activity occurring on premises or outside of a facility building is properly formulated and considered. Safety aspects of clients from third-party criminal assault must be weighed and considered" (Herbert, January 1992, p. 23). These responsibilities make the need for developing and using injury precaution sheets and appropriate risk management procedures all the more necessary, especially in situations which could very easily be overlooked by program leaders and administrators.

Specialized Training

Program sponsors must be prepared for any type of emergency. Therefore, professional standards of care dictate that facilities involved in physical, recreational, leisure, sport, and related activities have individuals present who are trained and competent in procedures such as first aid, CPR, and the Heimlich maneuver (Herbert, July 1991).

The American College of Sports Medicine's *Health/Fitness Standards and Guidelines* were developed through consensus of professionals in health club operations and management, club associations, physicians, physiologists, and a lawyer. Each of 22 chapters is divided into a set of standards (expected conduct) and guidelines (recommended conduct), providing clear benchmarks of expected duty for health clubs and fitness facilities (Herbert, July 1992). For example, "All facility staff must be CPR certified"; and "A first aid certified staff member must be on duty at all time." Facilities must become familiar with what will be expected of them in their own operations and procedures as provided by the ACSM publication, which will undoubtedly become their expected standard of care.

Programs requiring highly specialized competencies (e.g., swimming and other aquatic activities, adventure and ropes courses, spelunking, mountain climbing) must have leaders with necessary background, specialized training, experience, and certification. To do less will not fulfill the appropriate standard of care expected for participants in such activities. Additional training for leaders and administrators is necessary in such programs so appropriate accommodations can be made for participants with disabilities.

Injury Precaution Sheets

The heart of an effective informed consent program is an injury precaution sheet. Simply discussing safety precautions, potential dangers of an activity, appropriate rules and regulations, or spotting requirements and procedures is not sufficient. Too often these topics are dealt with during the first class period of a unit, first practice session of a sport, or first meeting in a recreation program and seldom discussed afterwards, unless a participant is seen violating rules so an unsafe situation arises. Anyone absent at the time of discussion receives little if any information about safety for the activity or sport.

Usually at the first session, little opportunity is provided for discussion, questions from participants, or elaboration since both participants and leaders want to get into the activity. Parents seldom know potential dangers faced by their children in physical education, sport, and recreational activities. Responsibilities involved here are not different in programs and activities involving participants with disabilities.

Judgments of the Seattle Case have brought about many changes in expectations related to potential dangers in activities for participants. In addition to all procedures and approaches previously discussed, additional steps must be taken by teachers, coaches, and leaders so participants are more aware of dangers facing them and injuries are less likely to occur. Well-planned and developed injury precaution sheets (see Appendix 1 and Appendix 2 at the end of this article for practical examples from public school swimming and lifeguarding programs) can include but are not limited to:

- Possible injuries, including those of a catastrophic nature, and how each can occur.
- Rules of play providing information and interpretations about rules with particular implications for safe participation.
- Safety rules to provide maximum safety for all program participants.
- Safety equipment and its use to guard against personal injury.
- Skill performance and instructional progressions as each relates to safe participation.

It is a good idea to have program participants sign a copy of the injury precaution sheet. This document should ideally be no more than one page and at most front and back of one sheet. Parents or guardians should have opportunities to review them, discuss them with their children, and return signed copies indicating they have seen and reviewed them. This is especially necessary when parents are actually ones assuming risks for their child's participation.

Injury precaution sheets are necessary for every activity and sport, not just those perceived to be of high risk. With each new unit, sport, or activity, an injury precaution sheet should be developed, distributed, and discussed. This procedure should be supplemented in various ways, including:

- Show various audiovisual presentations such as *Informed Consent* (1983) or *Warning: It Could Happen to You* (n.d.) with appropriate discussion and follow up.
- Use special stickers on equipment warning of dangers to participants, especially if these devices are used improperly or inappropriately. Obtain readily obtainable stickers for equipment for which they are available, or make your own when and where needed.
- Include as topic in meetings with parents or guardians, such as preseason for sport, back-to-school night, PTA gatherings.

All factors just discussed are appropriate and applicable when dealing with program participants possessing disabilities, whether in integrated or segregated settings. However, specific considerations related to an individual's disability and its implications for safe participation must be included in injury precaution sheets developed for these individuals. Major emphasis must be on ways a disability affects an individual's ability to learn and participate in activities. Obviously, implications and cautions related to potential dangers of actual medical conditions in these activities must be included. Not only must content deal with implications of the condition related to the specific activity, but means of presentation must be appropriate to the condition of the individual.

Following are additional representative, but not all-inclusive, factors to consider when developing injury precaution sheets to be used with program participants possessing disabilities:

- Medical factors as appropriate and necessary.
- Ways conditions affect an individual's ability to learn and participate in physical, recreational, leisure, sport, and related activities.
- Instruction/supervision.

- Assistance by and roles of peer participants, caregiver helpers, instructor, and instructional aides.
- Rule modifications and accommodations.
- Integrated and segregated settings.
- Means of presentations (creative, resourceful; language, terminology).
- Attention to environment itself—sound for deep end of swimming pool; visual warnings for hearing impaired; overall facility lighting.
- Adapted equipment.
- Class size.
- Level of activity/risk.

Contents of injury precaution sheets must be presented, discussed, and reviewed with program participants; they must be emphasized during instruction, practice, and participation/play times. Specific consideration must be given to these presentations when individuals with disabilities are among program participants. For example:

- Have injury precaution sheets in large print, braille, and/or audiocassette formats (only about 10 to 15% of individuals who are blind read braille) for use in and out of class by students with visual impairments.
- Use some form of sign language and visual supplements, including captioned videotapes, to augment oral presentations for students who have hearing impairments. Develop with your students signs for use in your own classes. Be sure students with hearing impairments are positioned in appropriate places in front of the class where they can see you and more accurately speech read.
- Develop special materials and presentations for use with individuals with cognitive conditions (mental retardation, learning disabilities)—e.g., use more basic vocabulary, keep on their level of understanding; develop visual supplements with graphic materials, slides, and/or videocassettes; turn sound track off regular films and video presentations, and do your own narration; make applications as practical as possible for individual program participants; use a great deal of repetition.

Parting Thoughts

Well-planned and implemented risk management programs, including injury precaution sheets, are not going to prevent either accidents or law suits. However, they will enable students, athletes, and other program participants to take part in overall safer environments and situations. Program participants will be more aware of dangers in each activity and know how to participate in safer and saner ways and how to protect themselves and their opponents from unnecessary and unwarranted dangers.

Administrators, teachers, coaches, and program leaders must know their activities, including inherent and potential catastrophic dangers. They must know how to prepare program participants to protect themselves. Individuals entrusted to our care can expect such preparation to protect against dangers. To do less is to shirk our professional obligations and moral responsibilities.

Selected References/Resources

Adams, Samuel H. (1982). Court decision hits hard with new liability twists. *Athletic Purchasing and Facilities*.

Adams, Samuel H. (1985). Implications of the Seattle decision. In *Sports and Law: Contemporary Issues*, Herb Appenzeller (Ed.). Charlottesville, VA: Michie Company.

Adams, Samuel H., & Mary Ann Bayless (1982). How the Seattle decision affects liability and you. *Athletic Purchasing and Facilities*.

Appenzeller, Herb (1978). *Physical education and the law*. Charlottesville, VA: Michie Company.

Dauer, Victor P., & Robert P. Pangrazi. (1989). Legal liability and proper care of students. In *Dynamic Physical Education for Elementary School Children*. New York: Macmillan Publishing Company.

Herbert, David L. Law Notes. *Fitness Management*.
Can GXTs be deemed "inherently dangerous?" Vol. 7, No. 7 (June, 1991), p. 29.
"Dangerous" bike costs a half million dollars, Vol. 8, No. 2 (February, 1992), p. 18.
Death in club whirlpool results in litigation, Vol. 8, No. 6 (May, 1992), p. 22.
Do clubs owe a duty to render first aid or CPR? Vol. 7, No. 8 (July, 1991), p. 23-24.
Equipment endangers unsupervised children, Vol. 6, No. 13 (December, 1990), p. 23.
Husband's release does not bar wife's lawsuit, Vol. 8, No. 7 (June, 1992), p. 22.
New standards for graded exercise testing, Vol. 7, No. 5 (April, 1991), p. 42.
New standards for testing and prescription, Vol. 8, No. 5 (April, 1992), p. 16.
Outside activities pose special concerns, Vol. 7, No. 9 (August, 1991), p. 26.
Owner not liable in use after closing time, Vol. 8, No. 1 (January, 1992), p. 23.
Participant release may leave spouse free to sue, Vol. 7, No. 1 (January, 1991), p. 19.

Personal fitness training standards, Vol. 8, No. 4 (March, 1992), p. 27.

Prospective release bars $ million jury verdict, Vol. 7, No. 13 (December, 1991), p. 24.

Standards for clubs now "the law," Vol. 8, No. 8 (July, 1992), p. 19.

Supervising children in the health club, Vol. 7, No. 12 (November, 1991), p. 26.

Use of weight-loss release upheld, Vol. 7, No. 6 (May, 1991), p. 22.

Informed consent (1/2" VHS video, 12 min.) (1983). Phoenix, AZ: Universal Dimensions, Inc.

Stein, Julian U. (1991). Injury precaution sheets: You can't afford to be without them. *Journal of the Virginia Association for Health, Physical Education, Recreation, and Dance,* April 1991 (13:2), reprinted with permission in *Indiana Journal of Health, Physical Education, Recreation, and Dance,* Spring 1991 (20:2).

Turner, Robert B. (1986). Failure to warn. *Virginia Journal for Health, Physical Education, Recreation, and Dance.*

U.S. House of Representatives (1990). Americans with Disabilities Act of 1990: Conference Report. 101st Congress. 2nd Session, Report 101-596; July 12.

Warning: It could happen to you (16mm, sound, color, 13 min.) (n.d.). Cedar Rapids, IA: Triad Films.

Zambito, Thomas (1992). Sports waivers worthless: State court rules injured man can recover damages. *Fairfax Journal,* June 10, 1992, p. 1.

APPENDIX 1

Swimming Safety Procedures

Read Carefully

The swimming pool can be a fun place. Many new skills can be learned and your body can get much beneficial exercise. However, the swimming pool is also a place where you could become seriously injured, or die! The following safety procedures are for the welfare of all swimmers. Read them carefully. You will be expected to follow these procedures when in the pool area. You will have a written test on this material.

Before Entering the Pool

1. Walk at all times when moving through the shower room and onto the deck area. The floors are wet and can be slippery. A fall can cause broken bones and other serious injury.
2. Shower and put on your cap before entering the water. A clean pool is important to your health. Help us keep it that way.
3. Check your body for any open sores. You will be excused until they heal. Open sores spread bacteria.

Entering the Pool

1. Always enter the water by sitting down and sliding in over the side. Jumping in and diving in are not allowed in the shallow end of the pool. They are allowed in the deep end—only at a designated area.
2. Diving is only allowed at a specific area of the deep end. Diving in when the water is too shal-

low, or when other swimmers are near, can cause spinal cord injury resulting in permanent paralysis or death.
3. The diving blocks are off limits. No student is to be on the blocks at any time.
4. When diving from the deck, you must be facing forward (no back or turning dives). It must be a standing dive. You may not run and dive from the deck. Before diving, be sure no swimmer is in the diving area.

Swimming

1. To swim in deep water, you must pass a deep water test. Do not cross the life line or go beyond water that is chest deep if you have not passed this test. You could drown.
2. Be courteous to other swimmers. No splashing, dunking, grabbing, or carrying of other swimmers. Keep your hands to yourself.
3. Wear your cap at all times. If it comes off while swimming, put it back on as soon as possible.
4. Look where you are going. Collisions can cause serious injuries.
5. A whistle means STOP, LOOK, AND LISTEN IMMEDIATELY. You or someone else may be in danger.
6. Exit the pool promptly when asked to do so.
7. If you are not swimming on a particular day you must bring a written excuse. If you need to be excused for more than a few days, a doctor's excuse may be required. You will be given an alternate written assignment.

These procedures were developed and used by Susan J. Grosse,
Milwaukee School of the Arts, Milwaukee, Wisconsin.

Swim Safety Procedures Test

Section One—True or False

To be considered true, a statement must be true in every respect. Read each statement carefully before you circle your answer.

T F   1. It is alright to dive head first into shallow water as long as you look first.

T F   2. You must pass a deep water swim test before you can swim in the deep end during free time.

T F   3. A whistle means that you should stop, look, and listen immediately.

T F   4. You can dive in anywhere as long as it is in deep water.

T F   5. Only people with hair longer than three inches must wear a swim cap.

T F   6. You could be killed or become paralyzed from going head first into water that is too shallow.

T F   7. Wrestling in the water is alright as long as both people agree to it.

T F   8. People who have passed their deep water test may go in the deep water as long as they hold onto the side of the pool.

T F   9. Only those students who have not had a bath in two days must shower before entering the pool.

T F   10. When the instructor tells you to get out of the pool, you have two additional minutes to play.

Section Two—Complete the Statement

For each statement, supply the most accurate words that will complete that statement (based on the swim safety rules).

1. Where are you allowed to dive into the pool?
_____

2. Two things each student must bring on swim days

are a _____ and a _____ .

3. When moving on the deck of the pool you should

_____ at all times.

4. If you cannot swim on any particular day you must

bring _____ and you will be re-

quired to do _____ .

5. An example of a serious diving injury that can

occur from diving into shallow water is _____

_____ .

6. A whistle means _____ , _____ ,

and _____ .

Lifeguarding—
Informed Participation

Sport injury liability litigation is on the increase. One determining factor in many court cases is whether or not participants were informed of inherent dangers of participation before initiating activity. Lifeguarding courses, because of physical contact involved as well as the nature of aquatic involvement itself, present a clear and present danger to participants.

The following information sheet is intended to inform potential lifeguarding students about these risks, as well as to make them aware of necessary safety precautions. Ideally this information sheet should be presented to each student before any instruction begins. Instructors should add to this information any data particular to their specific classes, including information on the lake or pool facility itself, particularly relating to water depth, use of a buddy system, handling specialized equipment such as a respirator, and rules for class organization and operation. Any student who fails to follow prescribed safety precautions of a lifeguarding course should be dropped from the course.

Lifeguarding
Injury Precaution/Information Sheet

Lifeguarding skills can be used in various aquatic environments, including indoor and outdoor pools and natural open waters, rivers, and lakes. Lifeguarding skills require both mental and physical abilities on the part of the participant at least equal to nationally established standards (American Red Cross, YMCA). The practice of lifeguarding involves contact with other individuals and, in the case of having to use actual life saving skills, physical contact with other persons has to be made. Such contact could be life-threatening to the rescuer, particularly if proper techniques are not used.

Anyone considering becoming a lifeguard, and/ or taking a training course in lifeguarding, should be aware that participation requires a high degree of personal fitness. Strength and endurance in executing swimming strokes (e.g., front crawl, breast stroke, and side stroke) are necessary, as is excellent breath control. Executing life saving techniques includes handling various types of land equipment and small craft and performing a variety of defenses, escapes, releases, and carries requiring body contact with another person, a person who may be panic stricken and completely out of control. Lifeguarding activity may take place in a physical environment where water, air, or weather conditions are hazardous to one's health if proper precautions are not taken.

Possible Injuries

Catastrophic injuries related to lifeguarding participation include:

- Loss of life due to drowning in the process of making a rescue.
- Spinal cord injury resulting from incorrect diving or surface diving techniques.
- Severe brain damage due to lack of oxygen, which could occur if the rescuer loses control of a rescue situation.
- Head injury as a result of being hit in the head by the gunnel or other part of a small craft during capsize practice or small craft rescue.
- Head injury as a result of being hit in the head by equipment during rescue practice.

These materials for lifeguarding were developed and used by
Susan J. Grosse, Milwaukee School for the Arts, Milwaukee, Wisconsin.

Severe injuries related to lifeguarding include:
- Severe muscle and/or tendon injury resulting from improperly executed body contact techniques.
- Severe bruises resulting from equipment and/or small craft handling during rescue procedures.
- Physical reactions to the environment such as reactions to pool, chemicals, lake plants, sun.
- Scratches, cuts, and bruises due to contact with other swimmers, resulting from failure to maintain proper spacing.

Minor injuries related to lifeguarding include:
- Muscle and/or tendon strains and ligament sprains resulting from improperly executed body contact techniques.
- Bruises resulting from equipment and/or small craft handling during rescue procedures.
- Physical reactions to the environment such as reactions to pool, chemicals, lake plants, sun.
- Scrapes, cuts, and bruises resulting from collisions with other swimmers or improperly executed body contact techniques.

Safety Rules

Procedures have been established to provide maximum safety for students participating in lifeguarding classes. Failure to follow safety procedures could result in catastrophic, severe, or minor injury. For safety:
- Enter the water only when directed to do so by the instructor.
- Participate in all warm-up activities requested by instructor. Failure to warm up properly can result in muscle/tendon/ligament injury.
- Practice all body contact techniques slowly, on land first, then in shallow water with a passive victim. Proceed to practice with an active victim and/or in deep water only when directed to do so by the instructor.
- A practice victim who wishes the rescuer to let go *for any reason* should tap or pinch the rescuer three times. A rescuer receiving such a signal should *immediately* break all contact with practice victim.

- Practice only under the supervision of the instructor or another certified lifeguard.
- Practice rescue techniques only with another lifeguarding class student, lifeguard, or life guard training instructor. Practice with an unskilled partner can result in serious injury.
- Allow sufficient distance from other swimmers and pool sides during all practice activities. Practice in a confined space can result in injury.
- When using small craft during capsize and rescue practice maintain a constant awareness of where the craft is so as not to be hit by a moving or tipping craft.

Safety Equipment

Various types of rescue equipment are utilized in the practice of lifeguarding procedures, including poles, rescue tubes, rescue buoys, shepherd's crooks, heaving lines, throwing ring buoys, back boards, rescue boards, masks, fins, and snorkels. All equipment should be kept in good repair and ready to use at all times.

When an item of equipment is used it should be returned to its specific location and secured properly. Any damaged equipment should be reported immediately.

Rescue equipment should never be used for play or any other use than that for which it is originally intended.

Skill Performance

Incorrect skill performance can result in serious injury and/or drowning. A practice victim should use the let go signal when a practice partner is in error. A practice rescuer should immediately let go of a practice victim when signaled to do so. A rescuer should perform all skills as specified by the instructor. Do not improvise or modify techniques to personal tastes. Such improvising/modifying could result in serious injury and/or drowning.

Employment

Most lifeguarding jobs require a minimum standard performance and/or certification for employment. Attempting to function as a lifeguard without having specific qualifications outlined by a national certifying organization can result in serious injury and/or death by drowning. Only individuals having *current* certification in lifeguarding should be placed in situations requiring the possible use of lifeguarding skills. Persons not having current authorizations should not assume lifeguarding responsibilities.

Section Two

ACCESSIBILITY AND PARTICIPATION

Play Spaces For All: A Photo Collage

Susan J. Grosse
David N. Reams
Barbara M. Moody
Delores Richmond
Todd Teske

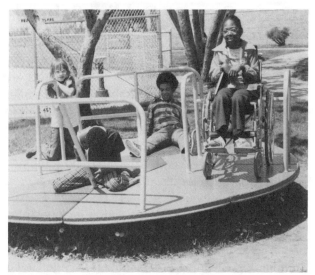

Individuals in wheelchairs need to play, too.

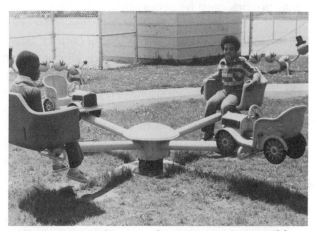

Different types of seats make equipment accessible.

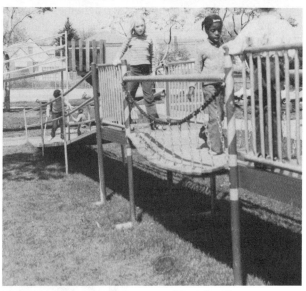

Play structures need ramps and hand rails.

All children have the right to play, but not all children are being allowed to exercise that right. In spite of repeated legislation mandating equal rights (including play rights) for individuals with disabilities and in spite of advances in the play equipment industry promoting accessibility, many playgrounds across the country are still not accessible to all children. Legislation does not, in and of itself, ensure change, nor does mechanical invention. People cause change.

This article is a photo collage of how people took the intent and concept of accessibility legislation, combined that with state-of-the-art possibilities in the playground industry, and created play areas accessible for all children, providing space for many different kinds of activities.

Accessibility means that individuals in wheelchairs can use the equipment. It means that different types of seats are available to make it it possible for individuals with differing balance abilities to participate. It means that there are ramps to allow accessibility for individuals with mobility impairment. And there are additional hand rails to provide assistance when needed.

If people set out to make a difference, play areas can be built and modified to allow participation by all children. This article presents examples of how three communities accomplished this task.

Dade County Public Schools, Florida

The goal of Dade County Public Schools is to foster integration of students with disabilities and students with no identified disabilities at the earliest age possible. To meet this goal, district standards for compliance with the Americans with Disabilities Act (ADA) of 1990 have been developed and implemented. With the exception of swings, no equipment will be approved for installation that will foster segregated play activities.

Title III of the ADA legislation includes playgrounds in those public accommodations that must be made accessible to persons with disabilities. The terminology defining accessibility is very general as it applies to playgrounds; however, it is clear that all playgrounds must be accessible.

The playground equipment options described in the following Dade County School District's standards for compliance with ADA are all composite structures. This does not limit single function equipment from consideration; however, it could not be approved unless its use was appropriate for children with disabilities or unless there were already accessible play structures located on the playground. When composite play structures are installed, it is not necessary for the entire structure to be fully accessible.

The minimum standards for accessibility are:

1. The structure must be ramped to at least one level and provide a minimum of two activities appropriate for children with disabilities. If less than two appropriate activities are available at that level, ramps must continue to other play stations until this minimum standard is accomplished.
2. Layered or tiered platforms may not extend more than two levels above the highest level accessible to children using wheelchairs.

3. On any play structure having one or more slides, at least one must be accessible to children using wheelchairs. Accessibility includes a transfer point from a horizontal platform large enough to accommodate a wheelchair and located 12 inches lower than the slide platform.
4. At least half of the stations, excluding upper-body devices, on each play structure must be accessible to children using wheelchairs.
5. Transfer points should begin with a platform 12 inches above the level accessible to a child in a wheelchair. Succeeding tiers should not exceed 8 inches in height.
6. Transfer platforms may be configured as squares, rectangles, or triangles.
   a. Squares must measure 4 feet on all sides.
   b. Rectangles must measure a minimum of 2 feet by 4 feet.
   c. Triangles must be right triangles measuring 4 feet along each arm.
7. The maximum height to be reached by transfer platforms when this is the sole means of access should not exceed 2 feet.
8. Ramps must be a minimum of 4 feet wide and a maximum of 10 feet long. The grade for incline ramps may not exceed 12 inches in 10 feet. A horizontal rest platform must be provided at a maximum distance of 10 feet on all incline ramps.
9. Ramps must be flushmounted to platforms. The entrance ramp should be flush at the 0 inch grade but must not exceed a 1/4 inch elevation above the grade.
10. Platforms must be a minimum of 4 feet by 4 feet. Except for ramped access points, all sides of each platform must be protected in a manner that will effectively and safely prevent junior size wheelchairs from rolling off the deck.

The photographs below and on the following page show examples of accessible play structures found in the Dade County Public Schools.

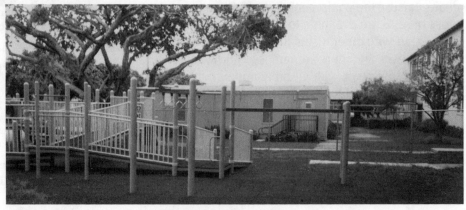

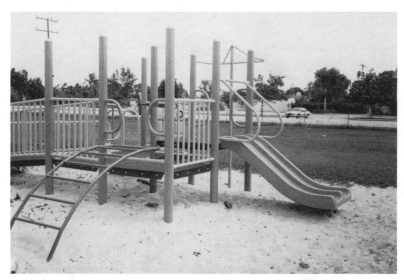

In the Dade County School District, at least one slide on a play structure must be made accessible to children using wheelchairs (above and below). Ramps must be a minimum of 4 feet wide and a maximum of 10 feet long and platforms must be protected to prevent wheelchairs from rolling off the deck (right). Dade County will not approve any equipment for installation if it fosters segregated play activities.

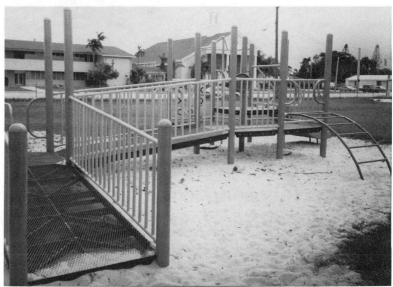

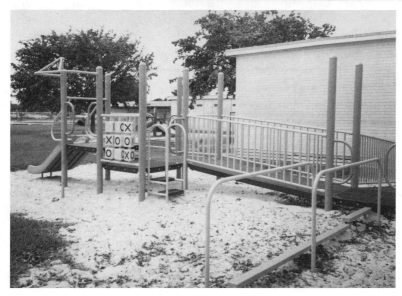

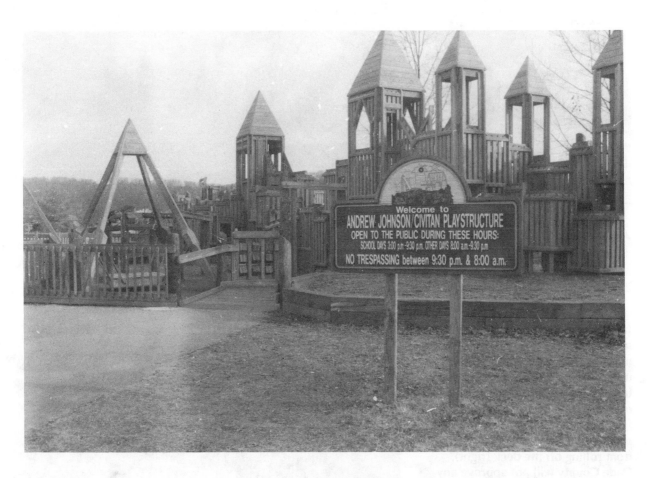

Andrew Johnson/Civitan Community PlayStructure, Andrew JohnsonElementary School, Kingsport, Tennessee

At the Johnson School, we worked through the PTA to build a Robert S. Leathers PlayStructure. Leathers' playgrounds are designed to suit the particular needs and dreams of the children who will use them. Incorporating ideas contributed by the children, each playground is a multi-leveled wooden structure with interconnecting tunnels, ramps, bridges, ladders, and overhead rings as well as sliding poles, slides, balance beams, and more. The structures are designed for continuous active play, to help children develop their upper-body strength, coordination, and both static and dynamic balance. They are also arranged to stimulate explorative and imaginative play, while at the same time leaving quiet corners where some children can sit and think, dream, or read.

Our playstructure has been designed to allow optimum play experiences for the disabled child as well as being stimulating enough to challenge even the most adventurous child. Dragons and castles, ramps and bridges, rings and tunnels all connect with an outdoor amphitheater. Children in all developmental levels will be able to play side by side and experience social interaction that might not ever be achieved in any other situation. The structure is 60% wheelchair accessible and 90% disabled accessible.

The Andrew Johnson/Civitan Community Play-Structure in Kingsport, Tennessee has become much more than the focal point for a child's free time during the school day. It's the answer to a classroom teacher's prayer. The play structure provides the ultimate in creative and developmental play, and also its design provides an outdoor classroom that can be used for anything from a nature lesson to the stage for a puppet show. The structure is the only one of its kind in Northeast Tennessee and is an exciting addition to the parks and recreation facilities for the Kingsport area.

Few of the nearly 2,000 volunteers who assisted in construction of the play structure understood that what they were building from scratch would provide for a child's needs in static and dynamic balance. Few perceived that gross motor skills for the disabled impaired would benefit. And even fewer had a clear idea of the playground's value for improving a child's social skills.

In a five-day span beginning on Halloween day in 1990, volunteers devoted their time and energy to chipping and cutting, bolting and securing the multi-level wooden structure. Civic organizations, volunteer pools, and skilled workers from industry and business, scouts of all ages, parents, teenagers, and members of the Army Corps of Engineers worked side by side. Numerous local businesses supplied building materials for the all-volunteer, built-by-donation playground.

When all was done, the school's PTA and area Civitan groups had spent an estimated $60,000 for a complex that is valued at $220,000. Based on the Robert S. Leathers PlayStructure concept, it extends a child's vision beyond traditional frolicking. It is a play structure that evokes self-reliance and team cooperation for participating children, as well as pride for the entire community.

Additional photographs of the community playstructure are on page 60.

The entrance (photo on page 58) to the Andrew Johnson/Civitan Community PlayStructure is from the school parking lot, which has wheelchair access. The actual area for individuals with disabilities portion is to the left and has a ground cover of Sportec. All children, regardless of ability, enjoy the creative, maze-like quality of the PlayStructure, pictured below.

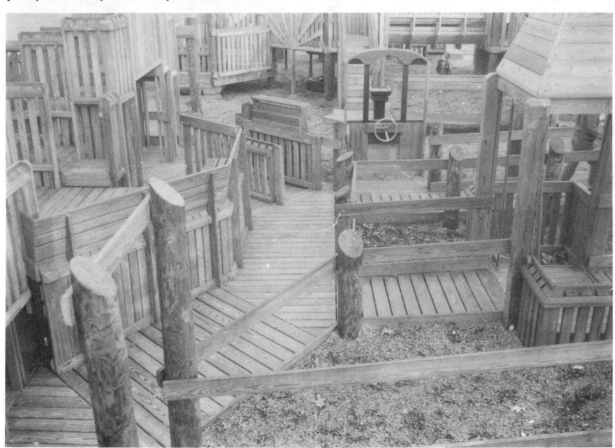

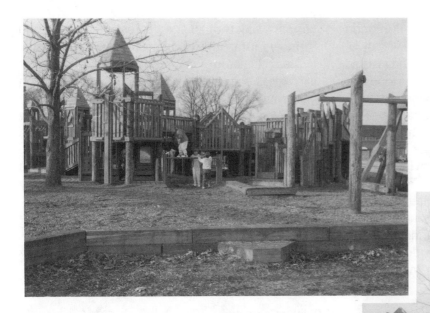

Depending on the disability, there are some portions of the structure (as shown above) that are inaccessible or only accessible with assistance. Wheelchairs move easily on all three surfaces: Sportec, wood ramps, and fibar (right). The opportunity for children of different ages and abilities to play side by side, to explore and to create makes the Andrew Johnson/Civitan Community PlayStructure a beautiful, magical place for activity.

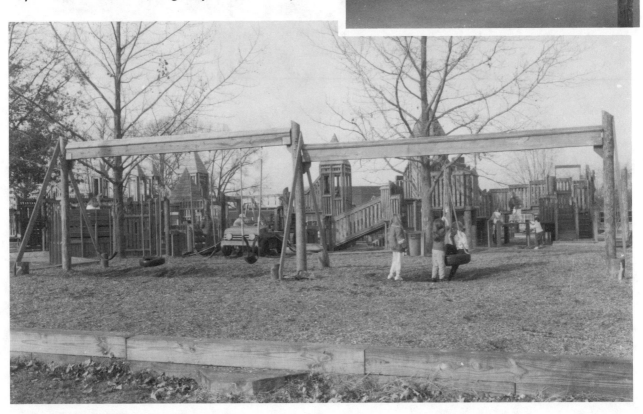

Eau Claire Barrier-Free Playground, Putnam Heights Elementary School, Eau Claire, Wisconsin

On August 26, 1990, the community of Eau Claire, Wisconsin, opened this country's first barrier-free playground with a new synthetic, padded surface. The project was funded through a federal revenue sharing funds grant; civic/service organizations; private, city, and in-kind contributions; a family foundation; and the public school district—a total community involvement. Major emphasis was placed on safety, integrational involvement, and low maintenance equipment. U.S. Consumer Product Safety Commission publications, *A Handbook for Public Playground Safety*, Vol. I and II and technical reports were instrumental in playground design/development. Additionally, assistance from the local technical college for drafting/mechanical needs was immensely helpful.

The funding was used to purchase adapted equipment, structures with ramp/handrails, paved pathways for wheelchair children, extra wide, double and enclosed slides, and swings that accommodate wheelchairs and children with lower extremity involvement. Additionally, a surface area was installed that absorbs falls and allows for accessible involvement, while meeting or exceeding all CPSC recommendations. This surface system involves an intricate layering of foam covered by outdoor carpeting. The "first-of-a-kind" surface in the United States allows for the safe utilization of wheelchairs, crutches, and other ambulatory equipment while maintaining a high degree of absorbency (shock absorption of 200g from a height of up to 10 feet 5 inches).

The specialized equipment was adapted into regular playground structures to ensure integration and appropriate development, socialization, and interaction for all children. Ramping allows for easy entrance and exit to various parts of the structure. Horizontal ladders and chinning bars are at wheel-

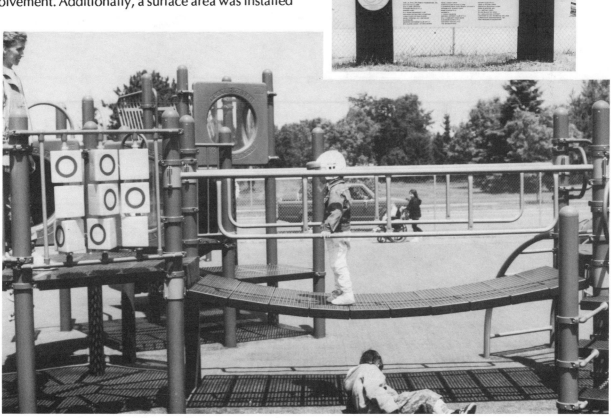

chair height. Slides are elevated to assist easier removal from wheelchairs. Dual slides allow aides to assist children as they go down. Posts are aluminum, and decks are rubber coated, heat resistant, and low maintenance.

The total cost of the playground was in excess of $86,000, not including construction, in-kind contributions, and discounts from surface and structure manufacturers. Other vendors contributed or substantially discounted their products for advertising purposes. Without such community and financial assistance, this project would easily have exceeded $150,000.

The playground is located adjacent to an elementary school with 400 students, of which almost 100 have exceptional educational needs. The playground is also used in the summer for the city's recreational program for individuals with disabilities. The main structure is completely modular so that if future expansion is necessary, it will be relatively easy.

Although "barrier-free" design increases the initial cost of facilities such as this one, the integrating benefits and opportunities are significant. The development of such projects needs to be encouraged.

Modifications and adaptations will certainly need to be made to assure continued safety. The benefits are overwhelming, and the time and effort put forth are certainly worthwhile in assuring that all children have equal opportunities. The community of Eau Claire, Wisconsin, is proud to have taken this initiative. The reward is ever so evident in the faces of all the children actively socializing and playing together.

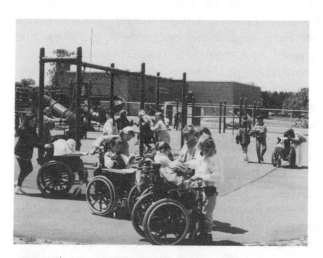

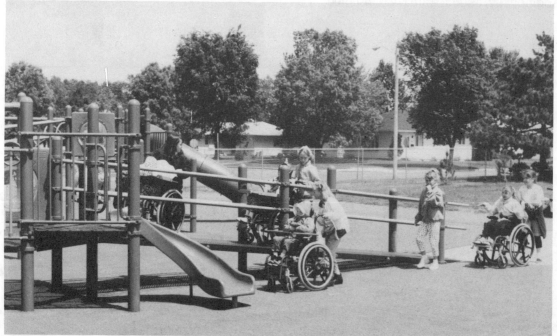

The absorbent synthetic surface (above) offers safety while permitting easy mobility for wheelchairs. The paved pathway around the playground area (top picture) allows for various activities and makes an easily maintained border for keeping debris off the playsurface. The clatter bridge with rigid railings (shown on page 61) permits balance opportunities for students.

Playground rules are posted on a sign with pictorial emblems (left). Specialized swings (below) permit individuals with lower extremity disabilities to experience appropriate physical development, as well as socialization and interaction.

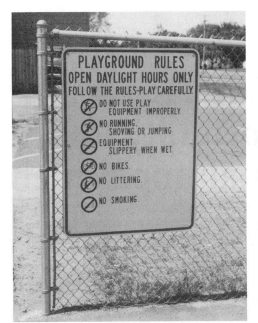

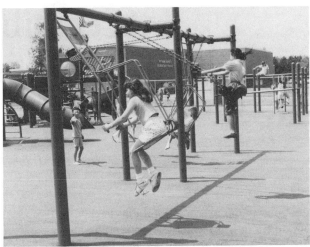

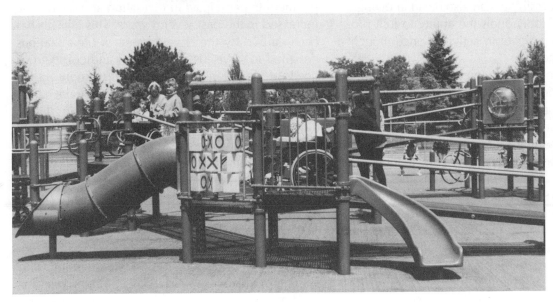

Various slides at wheelchair height permit easy transfer from chairs to slide. Tic-tac-toe panels allow the students to be active while waiting their turn.

For Additional Information

To learn more about these three facilities emphasizing accessibility for individuals with disabilities, contact the following:

David N. Reams, supervisor of physical education, Dade County Public Schools, Florida, 305-350-3011

Delores Richmond, principal, and Barbara M. Moody, physical education instructor, Andrew Johnson Elementary School, 1001 Ormond Drive, Kingsport, TN 37664, 615-378-8605

Todd Teske, coordinator of special services, Putnam Heights Elementary School, 633 W. MacArthur Ave., Eau Claire, WI 54701, 715-833-3421

Accessibility: Growth of Opportunity for Individuals with Visual Impairment

James V. Mastro

Accessibility means different things to different people. A curb-cut is great for someone in a wheelchair, but not for someone who is looking for the curb with a cane. Accessibility can also mean allowing a certain group of individuals the ability to join programs and to participate in activities once thought impossible for them.

Involvement in recreation and sport has been a part of the American way of life for many years. The need to participate is present in individuals with visual impairment, but they are likely to adopt a sedentary lifestyle unless they are given opportunities to be involved in and benefit from recreation and sport programs as early in life as possible (Buell, 1983; Mastro, 1985). Professionals in leisure programs have to increase awareness, eliminate myths, and provide legitimacy for individuals with visual impairment so they can bridge the gap from where they are now to where they should be in the future.

Realization of potential for individuals with visual impairment must come through education of significant others, such as parents, teachers, and coaches. Society in general must disregard perceived limitations and treat each as an individual with capabilities, emphasizing importance of training and hard work, without judging (Mastro, Hall, & Canabal, 1988).

Recreation and sport have social, therapeutic, and emotional value to individuals with visual impairment. In addition, they are of educational value, resulting in better understanding and improved relationships with the able-bodied community, aiding in an individual's adjustment, leading them away from social withdrawal and toward personal accomplishment (Lipton, 1981; Mastro, 1985).

Opportunities for individuals with visual impairment to participate in recreation and sport have increased in the past several years. This growth has been caused by the development of organizations designed to serve the recreational and competitive needs of individuals with visual impairment. However, leaders of these sport organizations have had to make do with limited resources and facilities, while their participants cry for equal opportunities to enjoy the privileges of programs for able-bodied individuals. Recreation and sport programs for individuals with visual impairment deserve the same amount and degree of financial funding as that provided by organizations for the able-bodied.

Monies should be appropriated for workshops and clinics, with opportunities for participation, development of new programs, and accessibility to existing programs emphasized. Clinics on coaching and training methods should be conducted by leaders in the field and athletes with visual impairment. Accomplishments of athletes involved in mainstream programs should be recognized.

Until recently, opportunities for individuals with visual impairment were limited because of lack of accessibility to facilities, adequate programs, rules, and technology. These factors affect the ability of individuals with visual impairments to determine whether they will be able to participate in recreation and sport.

Recreation and sport should be no different for individuals with visual impairment than for their normal peers. Overprotectiveness of these individuals by parents and specialists can cause more problems than the disability of blindness (Lambert & West, 1980). However, when there are individuals with visual impairment in recreation and sport programs, certain safety recommendations and considerations should be observed.

There are several important questions to ask:

What is the overall health of the individual with visual impairment?

- Does the individual with visual impairment have any other physical limitations (e.g., endurance, fitness, height, weight)? Check eye symptomology (e.g., eye imbalance or inflammation).
- What is the individual's visual acuity and field of vision?
  — Evaluate the individual's residual vision.
  — An individual with visual impairment may be able to watch a presentation if placed close to the front or if the demonstration is made to the good eye.
  — Make sure individuals who have glasses wear them.

What is the nature, cause, and prognosis of the individual's visual loss?

- Will their vision change with time (e.g., cataracts, glaucoma)? Some conditions may need environmental adaptations (e.g., intensity of lighting and use of incandescent light).
- Can vigorous physical activity further damage vision? Some conditions can be damaged by such activity (e.g., detached retina, diabetic retinopathy).

Is the individual's visual impairment acquired or congenital?

- If individuals have adventitious visual impairment after age five, they may be able to use visual imagery for movement they have never seen.
- Individuals with congenital visual impairment have to depend on other senses to learn movements (e.g., kinesthetic [the knowledge of body parts in space], tactile).

This article presents suggestions and considerations for specialists in recreation and sport, to help them understand the complexities of visual impairment and use correct methods in teaching. With this information, a safe and accessible recreation and sport program can become a reality.

Program Hints

A good recreation and sport program for students with visual impairment can be easy if common sense is used by instructors. Children need to experience fun and self-actualization, coming from successful interactions with peers and the environment. Specialists in recreation and sport use creativity, essentially treating individuals with visual impairment the same as normal students, to provide beneficial programs.

The following are hints to increase program participant success:

- Preschool and elementary children should be taught movement can be fun and beneficial, with some adaptations for safety. If you wait until these children reach 12 to 15 years of age, it may be too late for them to move with confidence (Buell, 1983).
- A good recreation and sport program can provide prerequisite skills needed for further participation in competition (e.g., increasing strength and flexibility).
- Use individuals with visual impairment during demonstrations of new movements.
- Choose familiar environments for physical activity or take time to orient individuals to their surroundings.
- Allow individuals to explore physical areas by themselves.
- Remove all obstacles that could interfere with free movements.
- Make certain activities are age appropriate.
- Make certain all adaptations are fair.
- Promote confidence and independence by letting children take risks.
- Use a radio or goal locators for cues in gym, playground, and swimming pool.
- Use aerial guide wires (e.g., guide ropes between poles), contrasting colors (e.g., between walls and floors), and textures as both visual and tactile stimulus for boundaries and for running.
- Use audible equipment or bright and contrasting colors (e.g., beep balls, balloons, scarfs, and goal locators).
- Attach bells to arms and legs of individuals to help them attend to their body position in space.
- Accentuate auditory attention to verbal instructions.
  - Emanate plenty of enthusiasm.
- Expand your verbal directions (e.g., "Go over there" is inadequate—where is there?).
- Provide verbal descriptions and manual manipulation guidance for instructions (e.g., braille).
- Adapt speed and length of presentations.

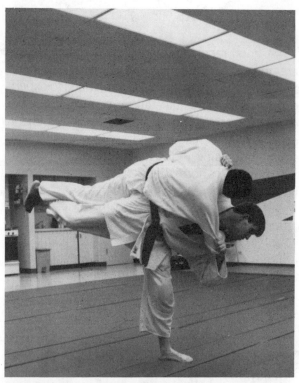

The United States Association for Blind Athletes has modified rules of various sports, including judo and track and field, to enable participants with disabilities the greatest degree of competition within a safe environment.

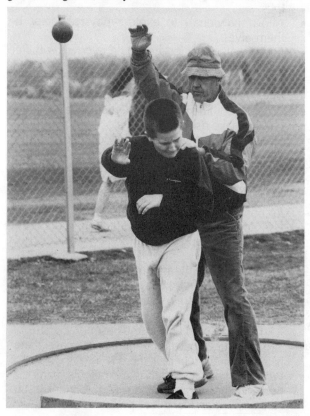

- Maintain normal voice intensity.
- Provide auditory starts and stops for activities.

These few hints will make your program more accessible and safer for individuals with visual impairment. Remember, these individuals have the same needs in recreation and sport as sighted individuals and you can help fulfill these needs.

Adaptations of Rules and Equipment

Rules for games are usually based on able-bodied sports, but adaptations can make games fair, challenging, and competitive for all players, according to the limitations of their visual impairments. However, recreation and sport should have no more modifications to the able-bodied competition than necessary at any level. If it does, questions can be raised as to whether it is an appropriate activity for integration (Nixon, 1989).

The United States Association for Blind Athletes (USABA) has rule modifications for such sports as cycling, gymnastics, judo, long distance and marathon running, power-lifting, swimming, track and field, wrestling, and the winter sports of Nordic and Alpine skiing and speed skating. Adaptations of these sports are made to enable participants the greatest degree of competition, within a safe environment (e.g., swimming—swimmers may use a bonker [a stick with a styrofoam end used to hit the swimmer on the top of the head before they hit the wall]; track and field—runners may use a guide; wrestling—competitors have a touch start).

Although the USABA has been developed for competition, one of their main goals is to make recreation and sport accessible to individuals with visual impairment. They play a role in encouraging specialists in recreation and sport to include students with visual impairment in mainstream programs, in elementary school, high school, or college. The USABA is working in conjunction with the U.S. Olympic Committee to make USOC National Governing Bodies accessible to qualified athletes with visual impairment (e.g., for athletes with visual impairment to qualify for the Paralympics, they have to participate in meets conducted by the National Governing Body for their sport). The USOC has been encouraging NGBs to provide athletes with visual impairment the sponsorship in developmental programs of their prospective sport and the resources needed to accomplish this goal.

Adaptation of Baseball

The National Beep Baseball Association (NBBA) has developed rules making our national pastime of baseball accessible to individuals with visual impairment. Certain rules have been adapted to make the game as safe as possible. However, it is not a game for individuals who are worried about bumps and scratches; there are some risks to playing beep baseball. Players dive on the ground to field a hit ball. A ball is fielded when it is picked up in hand off of the ground by a defensive player and an out is called by the umpire. Base runners go full speed to try to score a run. Players know there are risks but take them in stride because they want to play a game they love.

A game of beep baseball lasts six innings. Each team has three outs per inning. When a batter comes to the plate, one of three things will happen:

1. They will hit the ball and score a run.
2. They will hit the ball and be fielded out.
3. They will strike out (a strike out is four strikes rather than three).

The pitcher, catcher, and batter are all members of the same team. The pitcher tries to put the ball where the batter can make contact. A hit ball must go

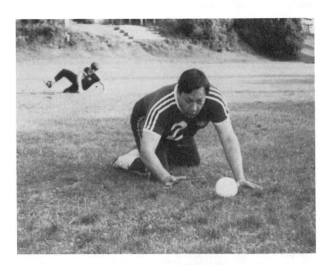

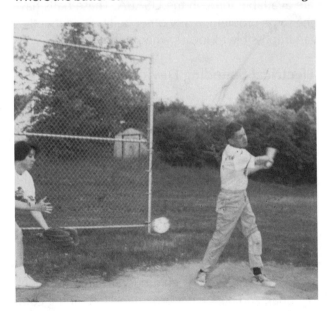

40 feet to be fair. There is no second base and first and third bases are 90 feet away from home plate and 10 feet outside of the foul line, to keep offense and defensive players from running into each other. The umpire determines whether first or third base will be activated. If the runner makes it to the buzzing base before the ball is fielded, a run is scored. If a hit ball strikes the pitcher, it is considered no pitch. Defensively, players can stand anywhere on the field. If a ball has been hit, one or two sighted "spotters" will call a number to tell fielders to what segment of the field the ball has been hit (the number three is usually center field). For safety's sake, they may also call "duck" if a ball is going to hit a player. Teams that have played together have very few collisions, but there is some risk.

Adaptation of Darts

The English Mark Darts Association, with the help of the Braille Sports Foundation, has developed rules and technology to make the game of darts accessible to people with visual impairment. Audio English Mark Darts is dependent on an electric "talking" dart board. A voice on the audio dart machine controls the game, providing all necessary information for playing (i.e., player number, round, when to throw, and who wins the game). Players must wait for the voice to stop talking before throwing a dart; the machine will not count a dart thrown while it is talking.

The game of darts has been made accessible to people with visual impairments.

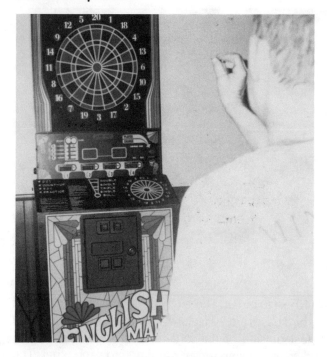

The only rules different from English Mark Darts are in the games of 301 and team 501. In 301, a player is limited to nine rounds (a round is three darts). If the player does not achieve a score of zero within nine rounds, the lowest score is the winner; 501 has a limit of 14 rounds (Ross, 1989).

Another modification of the machine is a roll-out carpet that indicates the throwing area. Eight feet from the board is the throwing line. It is a horizontal strip of wood with a notch in the middle, permanently affixed to the carpet. If a player needs assistance with balance, the back of a chair or walking aid is permissible. The Twin Cities Blind Audio Dart League has members who are not only blind but in wheelchairs as well. In tournament competition, all players wear blindfolds.

Technology

Individuals with disability have often benefited from technological advances and devices (e.g., motorized wheelchairs, electric doors, communication boards). Without these technological applications, accessibility is limited and opportunities to lead as normal and independent a life as possible are restricted. Individuals with visual impairment have benefited from technological gadgetries such as sonic guides and talking calculators, which increase their ability to participate in the mainstream of society. This section focuses on devices, such as audible equipment, that help make recreation and sport accessible to individuals with visual impairment.

Audible Balls

The most frequently used audible device is an adapted ball with a bell inside, and there are several types of bell balls, according to size, ranging in diameter from 4 to 13 inches (American Foundation, 1992). Individuals with visual impairment can track this type of ball when it is in motion, but cannot find it when it is stationary, making participation in certain activities difficult if not impossible.

Another kind of bell ball is the goal ball, made of a molded rubber substance with 8 to 10 holes and 5 to 7 ski bells placed inside. This ball was developed in Europe specifically for Goal Ball, a game invented after World War II to help rehabilitate war-blinded veterans. It is played on a field approximately the size of a volleyball court. A team consists of six players with three on a court at a time. The object is to throw-roll the ball past the other team's goal line. The game consists of two seven-minute periods with two three-minute overtime periods in case of ties. If the game still finishes in a tie, a one on one shoot-out is necessary.

Goal balls are not made in the United States but are available through the USABA. These balls have the same problem as any other bell ball, in that they are impossible to locate when stationary.

Electrical Sounding Devices

In 1964, Charles Fairbanks was given the task of designing a ball that would emit a sound, thus making games with a ball accessible to individuals with visual impairment. He inserted a small electrical device (beeper) into a regular softball, inventing the "beep baseball." With this ball and rules adapted by the Braille Sports Foundation in 1976, individuals with visual impairment were given the opportunity to participate in a form of our national pastime. The National Beep Baseball Association was founded later that year and has continued to conduct local, regional, and national tournaments, providing competition in a team sport for individuals with visual impairment (NBBA, 1991; Mastro, Montelione, Hall, & Richardson, 1987; Montelione & Mastro, 1985). (The game of beep baseball is described in more detail earlier in this chapter.)

The concept of a beeping ball was expanded, and electrical devices were placed in other types of recreational equipment, such as basketballs, nerfballs, footballs, volleyballs, and Frisbees. Problems with this equipment are that the devices are expensive and are not able to withstand heavy use. Often, balls with electrical beepers break down even with minimal use, thus spoiling fun and interrupting competition. The big advantage in using the beeping balls, however, is that the ball continues to beep after it has stopped moving.

Goal Locators

Goal locators are electrical sounding devices that emit an audible tone at different frequencies (e.g., one every second, one every 20 seconds, or

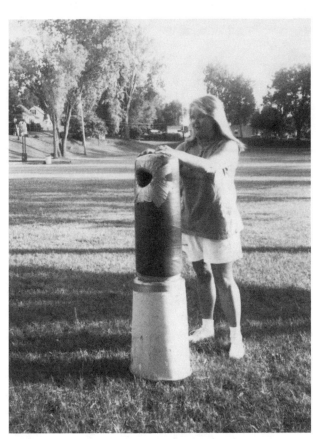

Goal locators that emit an audible tone can be used to mark any location for individuals with visual disabilities.

continuously). These devices are used to mark any location, such as a basketball hoop, a beep baseball base, or targets. The goal locator in basketball is placed on the back of the rim to let players with visual impairment know where to throw the ball. The beep baseball base, approximately 48 inches high, made of foam rubber and plastic, and shaped like a cylinder, contains an electrically powered sounding unit that emits a high-pitched tone.

Goal locators have been used for recreational games such as ring toss, bowling, and darts. The locator is placed on the post for ring toss, to mark the location of a headpin for bowling, and at the center of a target for darts (this is different from Audio English Mark Darts described earlier) (Reid, French, & Schultz, 1977).

Conclusion

Individuals with visual impairment have the right to enjoy the benefits of recreation and sport that may help them take their place in society. Even though it is difficult, they must be allowed to join the rest of the world and march to the same drummer. This inclusion in the mainstream must start as early in life as possible.

Much has been done to provide opportunities for persons with visual impairment in a wide variety of activities. This article could not, of course, mention all of the organizations that have developed programs, modified rules, and made technological advances, but all these additional opportunities contribute to accessibility into a normal life. Although much has been gained, more should be done to make existing programs accessible to individuals with visual impairment. Specialists in recreation and sport must use their creativity and initiative to make their programs accessible to all.

Organizations

American Foundation for the Blind (AFB) — 15 West 16th St., New York, NY 10011.

Braille Sports Foundation (BSF) — The goals and objectives of the BSF are to promote opportunities for persons with visual impairment to participate in therapeutic recreation and competitive sport. This is done by the bimonthly publication of *Feeling Sports,* clinics, and workshops given to educators, parents, and other organizations. Information on the National Blind Audio Dart Association (rules, games, how to purchase equipment) can also be obtained. To get on their mailing list or request a clinic or workshop, call or write James V. Mastro, BSF, 38-66th Way NE, Fridley, MN 55432, 612-574-9317.

LS&S Inc. — LS&S Group, P.O. Box 673, Northbrook, IL 60065.

National Beep Baseball Association (NBBA) — This organization promotes the sport of beep baseball. Information on rules, equipment, clinics, and workshops can be obtained by calling or writing Ed Bradley, President, NBBA, 9623 Spencer Highway, La Porte, TX 77571, 713-476-1592.

United States Association for Blind Athletes (USABA) — This organization is the National Governing Body (USOC) for sports for persons with visual impairment in the United States. A list of sports and rule modifications are found in the USABA handbook (approximately $3). Write or call USABA, 33 North Institute St., Brown Hall, Suite 015, Colorado Springs, CO 80903, 719-630-0422.

References

American Foundation for the Blind. (1992-1993). *Products for people with vision problems.* New York: AFB.

Buell, C. (1983). *Physical education for blind children* (2nd ed.). Springfield, IL: Charles C. Thomas.

Lambert, R., & West, M. (1980). Parenting styles and the depressive syndrome in congenitally blind individuals. *Journal of Visual Impairment and Blindness,* 74(9), 333-337.

Lipton, B. (1981). National Wheelchair Athletic Association and the Disabled Athlete. Presentation to the USOC House of Delegates, Colorado Springs, CO.

Specializing in products for the visually impaired. (1992-1993). Northbrook, IL: LS&S Inc.

Mastro, J.V. (1985). Diamond of the visually impaired athlete. *Palaestra,* 1(2), 43-46 (Macomb, IL).

Mastro, J.V., Hall, M.M., & Canabal, M.Y. (1988). Cultural and attitudinal similarities: Female and disabled individuals in sports and athletics, *Journal of Health, Physical Education, Recreation and Dance,* November/December, 80-83.

Mastro, J.V., Montelione, T., Hall, M.M., & Richardson, M. (1987). *Our noisy national pastime.* Macomb, IL: Palaestra.

Montelione, T., & Mastro, J.V. (1985). Beep baseball: What is it? *Journal of Health, Physical Education, Recreation and Dance,* August, 60-61, 65.

Nixon II, H.L. (1989). Integration of disabled people in mainstream sports: Case study of a partially sighted child. *Adapted Physical Activity Quarterly,* 6, 17-31.

National Beep Baseball Association. (1991). *The NBBA Guide.* Houston, TX: NBBA.

Reid, C., French, R., & Schultz, B. (1977). Use of an auditory cue to improve bowling performance of visually handicapped persons. *Perceptual and Motor Skills,* 45, 941-942.

Ross, J. (1989). A formula that works. *Feeling Sports Magazine,* Nov.-Dec.

To Give Them Roots and Wings
Re-exploring Accessibility Issues for Deaf and Hard-of-Hearing Program Participants

Ann E. Graziadei

Providers of programs for individuals with disabilities, both educational and recreational, have recently been forced to re-examine issues related to program accessibility. With passage of the Americans with Disabilities Act (ADA) and the Individuals with Disabilities Education Act (IDEA), program planners must examine their facilities and program offerings to determine compliance with these new statutes. Adapted physical education and therapeutic recreation professionals in professional preparation programs will also need to examine their programs as they teach future and practicing professionals to provide appropriate services to individuals with disabilities.

This article presents practical ideas regarding program accessibility for deaf and hard-of-hearing participants. These suggestions come from review of recent physical education, adapted physical education, and recreation literature and from colleagues and students in the Department of Physical Education and Recreation at Gallaudet University.

Professional preparation literature is straightforward regarding suggestions for handling deaf students in programs. The literature emphasizes integration with hearing peers, with the highest priority being promotion of social interaction; it strongly emphasizes that teachers and recreators should model the skills being taught and reinforce and encourage speech production (Auxter & Pyfer, 1989; Dauer &

Pangrazi, 1992; Horvat, 1990; Sherrill, 1986; Thomas, Lee, & Thomas, 1988; YMCA, 1987).

Interestingly, modeling, speech production, and social interaction are not the same issues raised by Gallaudet colleagues or students when they discuss program accessibility. Thus I would like to offer an alternative examination of issues impacting on safety and programming for deaf and hard-of-hearing participants.

In this brief article, I can only hope to make sense of a few points. First, I have chosen to examine recent literature and its emphasis on what should be taught and specific suggestions about including deaf and hard-of-hearing students in programs. Then I will identify what appears to be a major conflict within the literature. Third, I offer some observations about the creation, sources, and continuance of the conflict and suggest possible solutions. Finally, I offer some practical pointers for increasing program accessibility for participants who are deaf or hard-of-hearing.

Examining the Literature

Much of the knowledge base in adapted physical education and recreation is rooted in regular physical education teaching methodology. Various authors emphasize that general goals and objectives of physical education programs should focus on developing positive attitudes as well as a wide variety of skills and knowledge, resulting in a skillful and knowledgeable mover who continues to participate in activities throughout his/her lifetime (e.g., Kirchner, 1992; Nichols, 1990; Pangrazi & Dauer, 1992; Thomas et al., 1988).

Pedagogical literature emphasizes the need for a bias toward teaching knowledge, strategies, and safety-related information. Teaching such information assists students to become performers who incorporate a cognitive knowledge base to guide performance (Kirchner, 1992; Nichols, 1990; Pangrazi & Dauer, 1992; Pangrazi & Darst, 1991; Thomas et al., 1988; Vickers, 1990; Wall & Murray, 1989).

Imbedded in cognitive knowledge is the understanding that instruction includes teaching and practicing safely. Nichols reinforces this by stating that rules of safety should be established and communicated so that students are not asked to take unreasonable risks. Pangrazi and Dauer support this view by acknowledging the potential for injury in sports participation and state that safety procedures and simple first aid techniques should be taught.

Also addressed in the teaching methods literature are the negative effects of the "recreational approach" to teaching physical skills. Letting students play without an instructional focus allows the more skilled performers to become better while poorer performers do not improve and may actually suffer skill decrements because play is dominated by the more skilled players (Pangrazi & Dauer, 1992).

Thus the literature suggests that goals of instructional activity programs should focus on more than skill production. The cognitive knowledge portion of an activity should be equally emphasized because such knowledge contributes to understanding how to appropriately and safely participate.

The literature in adapted physical education and recreation offers similar thoughts regarding objectives of physical education for hard-of-hearing and deaf children. Auxter and Pyfer state that objectives of a physical education program for hard-of-hearing children are the same as those for nonhearing impaired children (1989, p. 288). They also state that the priority in physical education programming and instruction should be social interaction with hearing peers. This emphasis on programming for social interaction is also supported by Horvat and Sherrill.

A similar focus is suggested in several elementary and secondary physical education methods texts in their chapters about teaching elementary children with disabling conditions (Pangrazi & Dauer, 1992; Pangrazi & Darst, 1991; Thomas et al., 1988).

The literature also strongly suggests that modeling and visual clues are the best medium for communicating information about skills to deaf students. Auxter and Pyfer suggest that teachers should primarily focus on visual and kinesthetic skill instruction as this is what deaf people will rely upon.

When discussing skill production by deaf students, Horvat suggests that students may be deficient in motor functioning since they may not understand the rules and strategies of a particular game or sports activity (1990, p. 159). Sherrill suggests that as activities and games become more complex, deaf children do not grasp the intricacies (i.e., strategies and rules) of team games that are visually acquired in spontaneous play because they have had fewer opportunities for participation (1986, p. 572).

Conflicts Within the Literature

The information presented by the adapted physical education and recreation texts appears to me to be in conflict with itself and with the goals and objectives in physical education methods and materials texts. Goals of physical education in the methods texts strongly suggest that the program should be a well-balanced offering of opportunities to expand students' social, cognitive, and psychomotor skills. However, the adapted physical education texts suggest another agenda, one focused on social interaction but one that actually becomes social proximity or physical integration only.

What are deaf children in activity programs actually getting? They are often able to perform discrete skills such as dribbling, kicking, and striking. Many are able to participate in team and individual sport activites. However, these students often lack the ability to connect the proper name of the skill with the skill itself. Deaf students may be able to mimic the skill and perform it correctly but cannot identify when and under what conditions the skills should or should not be performed.

What the present physical education and recreation system has prepared, and is presently preparing, is a group of deaf and hard-of-hearing participants who are average participants but who do not have an adequate knowledge base. This is not a cognitive deficit of deaf and hard-of-hearing participants but rather a deficit in the instructional methodology presented in the literature that suggests instructors need only model the skills and face the students when they speak. Any sign language that is presented focuses on survival signing without regard to sending information about why, when, and where to perform the skills being taught.

The comments of Gallaudet students support this. The students questioned were taking an elementary physical education methods course, and they were all graduates of mainstream physical education programs in school. These are their thoughts about their past experiences.

Student #1

"What I can remember is that although I participated in PE activities, I didn't really understand what was going on because I didn't have my interpreter with me. PE was considered an 'easy' course so I didn't need an interpreter. I depended on my friends to fingerspell for me. I thought the PE program wasn't that bad or that great, just satisfactory. My skills and participation were average ... but my leadership wasn't. I never got picked as captain for a team, probably just because I was deaf."

Student #2

"For six years I had attended the public school which actually provided a program for the deaf. All of us, the deaf children, were integrated in the physical education program with hearing children. Of course, no interpreting was provided to us in the physical education program. As I recall, there were many various games and activities which did involve us.... The most essential activity of the physical education program was Field Days. It was an occasion in which every student participated in order to compete with each other."

Student #3

"I always struggled with 60s [grades in the 60s]. I rarely participated in class for fear of being laughed at because I 'misunderstood' the question. But when the time to go outside came, the teacher was able to see my other skills, or those skills I rarely used."

Student #4

"I don't remember much of my elementary school time. I was mainstreamed in a public school in Tennessee. I remember my high school PE class better — again I was mainstreamed and had no interpreter.

"It's funny, I remember taking advanced lifesaving in high school. I was a strong swimmer and I copied everything. I passed with flying colors and got my advanced lifesaving certificate. I was really proud. I took it again and passed in the community college — again I had no interpreter.

"Then I got to Gallaudet and took advanced lifesaving. Boy, what a shock. I never realized how much I had missed. I knew all the skills from high school, but I didn't know when to use the skill. I finally learned all the names for the skills. I wish I knew this in the earlier classes."

What does this say about these students' physical education programs? I would suggest it sends a message saying that their schools do not value physical education. When no interpreter is provided, it suggests the material is not worth understanding. It also forces deaf students to work twice as hard to try to understand the information being spoken.

One of the myths and stereotypes related to deafness is that most deaf people are good lip readers. Actually, the understanding rate for those dependent on speech reading (lip reading) alone is approximately 20%–30%. Additionally, speech reading is often easier for those who became deaf after they learned the English language (Kaplan, Bally, & Garretson, 1987).

What is it we teach in physical education and recreation programs? I would suggest we teach safety and health-related fitness—things that cannot be adequately mimicked or taught kinesthetically. Several examples of things that cannot be mimicked come quickly to mind:

- Understanding how to lift in order to protect our backs from injury.
- When and when not to attempt to help a person in first aid, water safety, and lifeguarding courses.
- How to appropriately "spot" another performer (gymnastics, stunts, and self-testing activities).
- When and how to take resting, during, and post-activity heart rates and how to calculate target heart rate.
- When, where, and how to move safely in and around the water.

Thomas (1989, as cited in King, 1991) offers a salient observation that applies when considering the four students' experiences quoted above. He states that "Currently, deaf children in the United States are being educated NEAR hearing children rather than

WITH them, in pockets of isolation called self-contained and mainstream classroom" (p. 20).

Compare the comments of students #1, 2, 3, and 4 with this narrative from another student.

Student #5

"My elementary experience in physical education was fantastic and motivating. My school was public but I didn't mainstream with hearing students. I had a deaf program designed with three classrooms where the teachers talked and signed at the same time.

The elementary PE program was organized and planned very well, especially for the deaf kids. I enjoyed my elementary PE program very much. The program was creative. I was motivated and eager to come in the PE program and learn many new things. I had a lot of fun when I challenged myself and I learned a lot about myself."

The difference in student #5's experience was that her physical education teacher signed—and signed effectively. He was not just trained in "survival signs" in physical education, but was a competent signer. He was a teacher who was able to convey cognitive information about the knowledge base. Student #5 participates on several sports teams at Gallaudet and is actively involved in her physical education major classes. She is one of the better students in the major and possesses better background knowledge than many of the other students.

Sources of Solutions to the Conflict

Potential solutions to the conflict can be drawn from literature on school to community transition and literature on communication and cognition. Freeburg, Sendelbaugh, and Bullis (1991) suggest that misunderstandings about communication abilities of hard-of-hearing and deaf students often create unrealistic expectations of how well these students understand speech. The authors state that communication problems often originate with untrained listeners/instructors.

Literature on cognition and deafness suggests that deaf and hard-of-hearing students have trouble with specific types of communication. LaSasso (1990) notes that deaf and hard-of-hearing students often have difficulty answering abstract question forms (e.g., who, what, where, when, and how types of questions). Such difficulties become handicaps for these students in both incidental (i.e., leisure and recreational play) and formal (i.e., classroom and instructional) learning situations.

Wood (1991) addresses the issue succinctly when he states it is entirely possible that deaf children experience developmental and educational delays not because they lack a language of thought but because hearing people find it more difficult to pass on their knowledge, skill, and understanding because of problems of communciation (p. 249). He goes on to suggest that the primary use of physical manipulation and modeling results in students who ask fewer questions, have less speculative and imaginative behaviors, and have a meager linguistic diet.

Thus, literature in this area suggests that program delivery to deaf and hard-of-hearing individuals be examined in regard to the quality of actual communication occurring in physical education or recreational settings. Program planners and instructors need to examine their own practices, as hearing people, and analyze whether they are choosing the medium that is most conducive to improving information gain by the deaf participant or just choosing a delivery system that is easiest for the hearing instructor.

Increasing Accessibility

To increase deaf or hard-of-hearing participants' accessibility to the cognitive knowledge portion of learning in physical education and recreation programs, the first salient issue to be assessed is the program planner's/instructor's knowledge about deafness, in general, and the deaf or hard-of-hearing participants being served, specifically.

Specific knowledge about the deaf or hard-of-hearing program participant might include:

- How the participant prefers to receive information
  — using sign language only (which type of signing: American sign language, cued-speech, signed English)
  — using speech-reading only
  — using a combination of sign and speech-reading
  — written information provided during the class
  — written materials that can be read prior to the class/program
  — via an interpreter

- What information the participant presently knows.
- What, specifically, does the participant want to learn (it should be noted that for students in an educational program the curriculum may be fixed so this is not applicable).
- How the participant will indicate that he/she does not understand or has questions about the material being presented.
- Whether the participant will be wearing a hearing aid during participation.

It is important that hearing students in the class understand about the deaf person's need to maintain visual contact with the interpreter and/or instructor. Also, since many hearing participants may not know much about deafness, instructors may find it advantageous to let the deaf or hard-of-hearing person share some information about what his/her needs are in order to learn the skills or information being presented.

Other suggestions for increasing accessibility to the cognitive knowledge portion of what is being presented include:

- Use a blackboard or overhead projector to record important points or new vocabulary.
- Consider using a flip chart (rather than blackboard) because it preserves information students can look at again at a later time.
- Provide new vocabulary and/or lecture notes in advance.
- If students take notes as part of the class, have someone else take notes and then give a copy to deaf or hard-of-hearing participants.
- Use a "flash card" approach to make certain students know the names of skills or concepts being taught.
- Use students as peer instructors, especially if deaf or hard-of-hearing students find a "peer" is easier to speech-read.
- Since much classroom instruction comes as a result of participant-generated questions, give deaf participants time to identify who is speaking and, if necessary, repeat or rephrase questions before answering.
- If using interpreter, talk with interpreter and share specific vocabulary (and meaning) prior to class.
- Seek captioned tapes/films that can be used in class or given to the student to take home and view (a list appears at the end of this article).
- If participants will be wearing hearing aids during participation, remove nonessential sources of noise as hearing aids amplify everything.
- Check frequently for understanding by asking "why" and "when" types of questions and looking at the student faces for quizzical or perplexed looks when presenting new information.

I do not believe transfer of cognitive knowledge from hearing instructors to deaf or hard-of-hearing students or participants is an unattainable goal. We, as professionals, should well consider and remember the motto above the little red schoolhouse in the foyer of the Kendall Demonstration Elementary School (the elementary school on the Gallaudet campus).

"There are only two lasting bequests we
can hope to give our children—
One of these is roots;
The other is wings."

Deaf and hard-of-hearing students and participants need to have the basic knowledge, the "roots," of physical education and recreation program activities. It is only after providing these roots that we can hope to give our participants outside opportunities to use their "wings" and benefit from what they have learned.

Resources

Captioning and Captioned Films

Modern Talking Picture Service, Captioned Films for the Deaf, 5000 Park St. North, St. Petersburg, FL 33709, 800-237-6213 (V/TTD). Films and videotapes on a variety of topics including education (health and physical education) and special feature/interest. Service is free.

National Captioning Institute, 5203 Leesburg Pike, Falls Church, VA 22041, 703-998-2400 (V/TTD). Films and videotapes on a variety of topics.

The Caption Center, 125 Western Ave., Boston, MA 02134, 617-492-9925 (V/TTD). Films and videotapes on a variety of topics.

Gallaudet Media Distribution, c/o Gallaudet University Library, 800 Florida Ave., NE, Washington, DC 20002, 202-651-5322 (V/TTD). Films and videotapes on a variety of topics for free loan or purchase.

American Red Cross. Contact your local Red Cross Chapter. Closed captioned videos on topics including first aid, CPR, spinal injury management, and water safety.

American Tobacco Institute, 1875 I St., NW, Washington, DC 20006, 202-457-4882. An open captioned and signed fire safety video, "Stop, Drop, and Roll," featuring a deaf family is available free.

Gallaudet University Department of Physical Education, 800 Florida Ave., NE, Washington, DC 20002, 202-651-5591 (V/TTD). A 60-minute aerobic workout videotape "Sign 'n Sweat" done using sign language, open captions, voice, and music. Cost: $33 plus shipping.

Gina A. Oliva, P.O. Box 3224, Laurel, MD 20709. A video "Shape Up 'n Sign" featuring herself and six children age 6-10 who teach the manual alphabet, numbers, and two upbeat fitness songs (done in sign and voice). The tape is in two segments and each includes a warm-up, two sign-along songs with aerobic movement, and a cool-down. Cost: $23 plus shipping.

Contact your state's residential school for the deaf. They may have a lending library of captioned films/videos.

Sign Language and How to Sign

If you want to take a class, contacts include:

> local colleges/universities/community colleges
> local recreation departments
> public schools (evening classes and continuing education)
> outreach programs from schools for the deaf
> churches having a deaf minister
> local hospitals offering continuing education
> local or state governmental agencies.

If you want to get a video lesson or course:

Gallaudet Media Distribution, c/o Gallaudet University Library, 800 Florida Ave., NE, Washington, DC 20002, 202-651-5222 (V/TTD). Videotapes available for free loan or purchase.

Gallaudet University Bookstore, c/o Gallaudet University, 800 Florida Ave., NE, Washington, DC 20002, 202-651-5380 (V/TTD). Videotapes on sign language available for purchase.

Sign Enhancers, Inc., 1320 Edgewater St., NW, Suite B-10, ASL Department UM1, Salem OR 97304, 800-767-4461. A 15-video American sign language lesson program. Tapes can be purchased singly or as a package.

Contact your state residential school for the deaf. They may have a lending library.

If you want to get a book:

Gallaudet University Bookstore, c/o Gallaudet University, 800 Florida Ave., NE, Washington, DC 20002, 202-651-5380 (V/TTD). Books on sign language and deafness, available for purchase.

Contact your local public library or library of any college or university.

If you want to get more information about deafness:

National Academy, Gallaudet University, 800 Florida Ave., NE,, Washington, DC 20002, 202-651-5096 (V/TTD).

National Technical Institute for the Deaf, Public Information Office, One Lomb Memorial Dr., P.O. Box 9887, Rochester, NY 14623-0887, 716-475-6824 (V/TTD).

Alexander Graham Bell Association for the Deaf, 3417 Volta Pl., NW, Washington, DC 20007-2766, 202-337-5220 (V/TTD).

National Information Center on Deafness, Gallaudet University, 800 Florida Ave., NE, Washington, DC 20002, 202-651-5051 (V/TTD).

U.S. Team—World Games for the Deaf, P.O. Box USA, 800 Florida Ave., NE, Washington, DC 20002-3625. Information on athletic competition for the deaf.

References

Auxter, D., & Pyfer, J. (1989). *Principles and methods of adapted physical education and recreation.* St. Louis, MO: Times Mirror/Mosby College Publishing.

Freeburg, J., Sendelbaugh, J., & Bullis, M. (1991). Barriers in school-to-community transition. *American Annals of the Deaf,* 136(1), 38-48.

Graziadei, A.E. (1991). Stories from the mainstream. Paper presented at the Eighth International Symposium on Adapted Physical Activity, Miami, FL.

Horvat, M. (1990). *Physical education and sport for exceptional students.* Dubuque, IA: Wm. C. Brown.

Kaplan, H., Bally, S.J., & Garretson, C. (1987). *Speechreading: A way to improve understanding* (2nd ed.). Washington, DC: Gallaudet University Press.

King, J.F. (1991). What is happening to deaf children?: The misinterpretation of P.L. 94-142. *Perspectives in Education and Deafness,* 10(2), 20-21.

Kirchner, G. (1992). *Physical education for elementary school children* (8th ed.). Dubuque, IA: Wm. C. Brown.

LaSasso, C. (1990). Developing the ability of hearing-impaired students to comprehend and generate question forms. *American Annals of the Deaf,* 135(5), 409-412.

Nichols, B. (1990). *Moving and learning: The elementary school physical education experience* (2nd ed.). St. Louis, MO: Times Mirror/Mosby College Publishing.

Pangrazi, R.P., & Darst, P.W. (1991). *Dynamic physical education for secondary school students: Curriculum and instruction* (2nd ed.). New York: Macmillan.

Pangrazi, R.P., & Dauer, V.P. (1992). *Dynamic physical education for elementary school children* (10th ed.). New York: Macmillan.

Sherrill, C. (1986). *Adapted physical education and recreation: A multidisciplinary approach* (3rd ed.). Dubuque, IA: Wm. C. Brown.

Thomas, J.R., Lee, A.M., & Thomas, K. T. (1988). *Physical education for children: Concepts into practice.* Champaign, IL: Human Kinetics Books.

Vickers, J.N. (1990). *Instructional design for teaching physical activities: A knowledge structures approach.* Champaign, IL: Human Kinetics Books.

Play in the Child Care Setting
Creating Opportunities for Preschool Children with Disabilities

Sue C. Wortham

Although extensive research on play of normal children has provided significant assistance in design of quality playspaces, obtaining comparable information about children with disabilities is more difficult. Less research has been conducted for these young children, and the characteristics of individual children with disabilities can be complex, unique, and not easily generalized to groups of other children.

Characteristics of children with disabilities are difficult to describe because of the varied connotations applied to terms used to define conditions. Frost (1992) has charted categories of disabilities and how each may affect a child. The categories of physical, communication, and development and learning disabilities are described in terms of problems they may cause for the child. Figure 1 contains Frost's explanation of disabling conditions. In addition, there are also differences among children who have similar disabilities. Each individual child experiences limitations in play differently.

Information about play of children with disabilities has been difficult to obtain and apply to provisions for play opportunities. Hughes (1991) suggests this confusion results from the varied purposes for conducting research, inconsistent definitions of play, differences in goals, methods, and professional backgrounds of researchers, and the multiple disabilities investigated. Also, the term "handicapping condition" was frequently applied to a variety of disabilities, making results difficult to interpret.

In spite of difficulties encountered in conducting and interpreting research on play of children with disabilities, there is some helpful information about how a disability affects the child's play. Play leaders and teachers can use available information to intervene and enrich the play of children with disabilities.

Developmental Play in the Presence of a Disability

Young children use play to gain control of their environment. Children with disabilities may have varied limitations on how they are able to use and master the world around them. Attention to these limitations can assist caregivers in enhancing development through play for children with disabilities.

Blind children enjoy playing; however, their fantasy play is less imaginative than sighted children (Singer & Streiner, 1966). Because they are not able to use visual cues, they may also lag in social play (Rogow, 1991). Frost (1992) suggests ways adults can help children with visual disabilities overcome their restricted interaction with the world and the difficulty they may experience in orienting themselves to space and time.

- Adults can provide assistance by planning play experiences. Play materials, equipment, activities, and playmates should all be considered.

Figure 1. Categories of Disabilities and Their Consequences

Category	Specific Handicaps	Social and Personal Consequences

Physical	Crippled
	Birth defects
	Blind and partially sighted
	
	Neurological disorders
	  Cerebral palsy
	  Epilepsy
	
	Health Impaired
		The child has problems with:
		Mobility
		Experiencing the world through all of his
		  senses
		Mastering his physical and human environments
		People who are too helpful or too demanding
		People who do not understand his difficulties in
		  gaining mastery over his world
		Isolation
		Diminished energy

Communication	Speech
	Deaf and hard of hearing
	
	Language disorders
	  of childhood
	Severe language delay
	Multihandicapped
		The child has problems with:
		Learning or using verbal symbols to think
		  and communicate about his world
		Dealing with academic learning which
		  requires the use of verbal symbols
		Isolation

Development and learning	Mental retardation Behavior disorders Specific learning disabilities	*The child has problems with:* Reduced interest in the world Difficulty in relating positively to children and/or adults Developing internal controls Failure to live up to expectations Rejection and isolation

Joe L. Frost, *Play and Playscapes*, Delmar Publishers, Inc., 1992, p. 296.

- Prior to play, adults can help children practice with materials or equipment to be used.
- Play settings should have sensory clues, such as different textures on walking surfaces, identifying play zones or experiences.
- Adult supervisors should support and encourage children during play activities, especially in developing strategies to enter social play opportunities.

Children with delayed language frequently exhibit symbolic play deficits (Lombardino, Stein, Kricos, & Wolf, 1986). These children engage in make-believe play, but it is less mature and has less variety (Hughes, 1991).

Children with learning impairment may exhibit similar limitations in that they engage in less cooperative make-believe play. However, if children with hearing impairment play in integrated settings with children without a hearing loss, play is more socially sophisticated.

Young children with motor disabilities may have difficulty in mastering play environments, particularly if physical environments have not been adapted to provide accessibility. However, their play needs are the same as those of children with no disabling conditions. Their play environments should include (Frost, 1992):

- Play structures that provide opportunities for exploration.
- Opportunities for fantasy and gross motor play.
- Opportunities for digging and gardening.
- Opportunities for sand, mud, and water play.
- Opportunities for animal care.
- Opportunities for carpentry.
- A wealth of loose parts to stimulate creative play.

Soft shapes and a matted surface encourage children to be involved in exploratory motor activity.

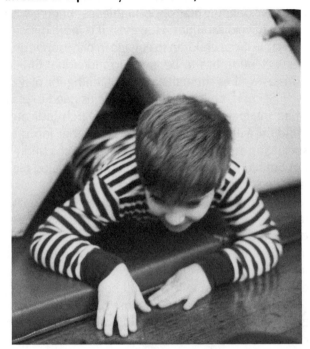

Children with physical disabilities may have restricted play behaviors related to accessibility of play experiences. Physical accommodation of play environments should make it possible to:

• Allow access to play experiences.
• Physically locate the young, less mobile children within a play experience, using adult assistance if necessary.
• Broaden opportunities for less mobile children to grow through play, while encouraging increased mobility.

Children with cognitive disabilities differ in intellectual as well as social play. They may not reach out and examine toys; they may be significantly delayed in exploratory strategies and symbolic play (Beeghly, Perry, & Cicchetti, 1989; Kopp, Krakow, & Johnson, 1983). A complicating factor is the possibility that their adult caregivers may underestimate their potential for play or have a feeling of hopelessness toward teaching play activities.

Children with cognitive disabilities can learn through play. Adult support might include:

• Facilitating social play through direct teaching and positive reinforcement.
• Using electronic toys with visual and auditory stimuli

to enhance the child's interest and help sustain play with objects (Frost, 1992).
• Adapting play environments to motor and sensory deficits of children with cognitive disabilities. Adult leadership is required to teach, prompt, and rehearse play behaviors (Strain, 1975).
• Integrating children with cognitive disabilities with higher functioning children. This may also increase their social play (DeVoney, Guralnik, & Rubin, 1974).

Children who are emotionally disturbed appear to fail to differentiate between themselves and the external world and may be unable to function within the social environment. They are more likely to engage in repetitive, stereotyped manipulation of toys. They rarely engage in symbolic play, and they lack the representational skills that can affect both social and symbolic play (Baron-Cohen, 1987).

Adult support to facilitate their play might include:

• Structuring social interactions so appropriate behaviors can be learned and positive results occur.
• Varying play equipment to avoid repetitive, stereotypic behaviors.
• Teaching new and specific play behaviors, particularly in relation to play equipment, to avoid repetition of inappropriate, previously learned behaviors.
• Providing immediate, positive feedback when appropriate play behavior occurs.
• Structuring play environments to focus the child's attention on the present, real world.

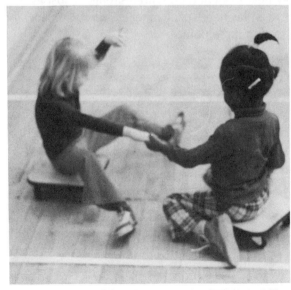

Using scooters for partner activities encourages mobility and increases social contact through problem solving.

Play Opportunities for Children with Disabilities

In the past there has been a low priority for play opportunities for young children with disabilities. Rising from perceptions of the needs of these children as they participate in segregated group settings and segregated preschool programs, emphasis has been on intervention activities to remediate developmental delay or individual limitations. Priority in these programs has been on direct instruction of specific skills, rather than on play. In many instances emphasis on teaching self-help skills has left little time for play. Parents of very young children with disabilities have often been hesitant to engage in spontaneous play because of the sometimes fragile condition caused by the disability. Some children are slow to respond to parents' attempts to play, and irritability and crying may discourage parents from engaging in playful interactions (Jackson, Robey, Watjus, & Chadwick, 1991).

When considering play opportunities for preschool children with disabilities there are several important points that must be addressed. First and foremost, child care settings are no longer segregated. Children with disabilities attend community day care along with their nondisabled peers. Commonality in grouping of children now comes from parent need for service, geographic location, and child age, rather than from presence of a disability.

All care givers should be prepared to address play needs of children with disabilities, just as they address play needs of all other children. Consider the following three points.

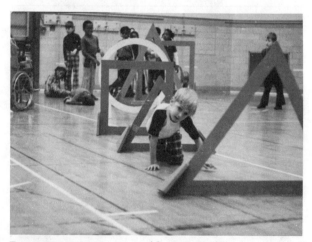

Day care centers must provide opportunities for play to all children, regardless of presence of disability

First, children with disabilities need to play; moreover, they can gain similar developmental benefits from ongoing play opportunities as children who do not have disabilities. However, it is more difficult to enable these children to engage in play opportunities. Attention has to be given to individual limitations as well as strengths, when planning for play.

Second, children with disabilities need to play in an integrated group. Because research indicates children with disabilities engage in higher forms of social and dramatic play when playing with children not limited by a disabling condition, integrated play is to be preferred whenever possible.

Also, many children with disabilities must be taught to play or prepared for play experiences. Peer children engage in play spontaneously without adult initiation. Children with disabilities may need adult instruction or intervention to negate limitations that prevent them from enjoying full benefits of play.

Special consideration must be given to play environments designed for children with disabilities. Planners at child care settings must consider unique disabilities or combinations of disabilities present in the population of children who will use the play environment, both presently and in the future. For example, accessibility considerations are different for young children who use wheelchairs for mobility compared to children who use walkers, crutches, braces, and/or canes. Children with visual disabilities need textural and auditory stimulation for play. Children with hearing disabilities need movement and visual stimulation to enhance play experiences.

Adapting Play Environments for Children with Disabilities

The Education for All Handicapped Children Act (P.L. 99-142), passed in 1975, mandated that all handicapped children, beginning at age 3, must be educated in the least restrictive setting. P.L. 99-457 extended intervention services to handicapped infants and toddlers. The Americans with Disabilities Act (ADA), P.L. 101-336, ensures that disabled persons will have access to public accommodations, businesses, and services operated by private entities. Play environments are considered part of the preschool child's least restrictive educational environment and part of the services provided by a child care center or other preschool setting.

In keeping with the intent of the laws regarding needs and rights of children with disabilities, outdoor playscapes at child care centers should allow for access by children with disabilities, whatever the disability may be. Raschke, Dedrick, and Hanus (1991) propose that "adaptive playgrounds should be designed for children who crawl, slide, or roll, as well as for those who walk and run" (p. 25). This statement can be expanded to include young children with visual, auditory, cognitive, or emotional disabilities.

When designing play opportunities for very young children, whether or not they have disabilities, their level of development and developmental needs are considered. Raschke, Dedrick, and Hanus suggest that playgrounds should be designed to:

- Encourage children to use all of their senses.
- Allow children to feel independent and improve their self-images by individually manipulating the environment.
- Foster communication and social contact with other children.
- Enrich gross and fine motor skills by providing a variety of activities requiring responses of varying degrees of difficulty.
- Provide a broad range of media to help develop cognitive skills.
- Promote an atmosphere fostering recreational and creative play. (p.25)

In *Play for All Guidelines* (Moore, Goltsman, & Iacofano, 1987), child development objectives are part of well-designed play environments, including opportunities for motor skill development, decision making, learning, fantasy play, and social development. More importantly, playing should be fun! To achieve a developmentally appropriate play environment adapted to children with disabilities, Raschke, Dedrick, and Hanus (1991) offer an instrument to facilitate a needs assessment for the design and construction of adaptive playgrounds (Figure 2, see next page). Although a few of the items on the survey are relevant for older children, most items are suitable for consideration for playgrounds for all children, regardless of age or disability, and can be readily used by child care centers.

Design and construction of a play environment usable by children with all types of disabilities is part of the process of providing play opportunities to ALL young children. The key to making play possible for very young children with disabilities is still adult care givers and/or teachers. Adults must assess the child's abilities and limitations in play and devise a plan to empower that child to make as much use of the play environment as possible. Adult care givers must enrich environments with materials and play opportunities, responding to needs of individual children with physical, social, emotional, and cognitive development in mind. They must be observers of each child's play ,and play for and with children to extend the range and enjoyment of play opportunities.

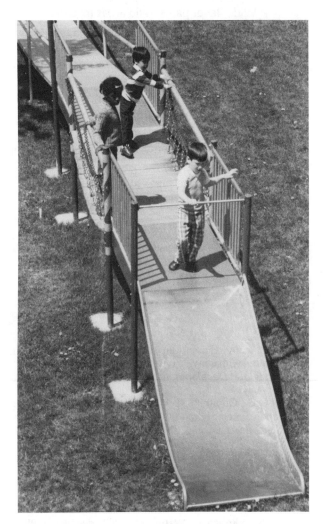

Playground equipment should be accessible to all children. Adding ramps and stability bars to this swing bridge and slide makes it accessible to children with physical disabilities.

References are on next page.

Figure 2. Adaptive Playground Needs Assessment

This survey is designed to determine your priorities for the design and construction of an adaptive playground. Using a scale of 1 to 5, give a 5 to your highest and a 1 to your lowest priority items.

The adaptive playground should include:

An area composed of cargo nets, ropes, etc.
A picnic area with tables, grass, bushes
Wide, level paths to tie areas together
A fenced playground with large gates
A structure with multiple levels for climbing
A sun-shaded outside classroom with seating
A horticultural center area
A quiet place for privacy — no intruders
A sheltered area with huge wooden boxes
A castle or other role-playing structure
Stationary wooden vehicles such as a fire engine
An area specially designed for crawlers
Huge concrete pipes to crawl through
A multiple-level playhouse

Traditional playground equipment with adaptations
   (e.g., slide with ramps)
An open area with movable cubes, boards
A large sandbox, sand tables
Water tables and outdoor water fountain
An outdoor ramp with rails
A stage area for play productions, singing, etc.
A balancing beam area
Boards with obstructions to crawl around
A permanent Special Olympics training area
A protected running track area
Towers with platforms, ladders, etc.
Tires to crawl through

D.B. Raschke, C.V.L. Dedrick, and K. Hanus, Adaptive Playgounds for All Children, *Teaching Exceptional Children*, Fall 1991, p. 26

References

Beeghly, M., Perry, B.W., & Chichetti, D. (1989). Structural and affective dimensions of play development in young children with Down's syndrome. *International Journal of Behavioral Development*, 12, 257-277.

Devoney, C., Guralnik, M., & Rubin, H. (1974). Integrating handicapped and nonhandicapped preschool children: Effects on social play. *Childhood Education*, 50, 360-364.

Frost, J.L. (1992). *Play and playscapes*. Albany, NY: Delmar.

Hughes, F.P. (1991). *Children, play and development*. Boston: Allyn and Bacon.

Jackson, S.C., Robey, L., Watjus, M., & Chadwick, E. (1991). Play for all children: The toy library solution. *Childhood Education*, 68, 27-31.

Kopp, C., Krakow, J., & Johnson, L. (1983). Strategy production by young Down's syndrome children. *American Journal of Mental Deficiency*, 88, 164-169.

Lombardino, L.L., Stein, J.E., Kricos, P.B., & Wolf, M.A. (1986). Play diversity and structural relationships in the play and language of language-impaired and language-normal preschoolers: Preliminary data. *Journal of Communications Disorders*, 19, 475-489.

Moore, R.C., Goltsman, S.M., & Iacofano, D.C. (Eds.). (1987). *Play for all guidelines: Planning, design and management of outdoor play settings for all children*. Berkeley, CA: MIG Communications.

Raschke, D.B., Dedrick, C.V.L., & Hanus, K. (1991). Adaptive playgrounds for all children. *Teaching Exceptional children*, 25-28.

Rogow, S.M. Dynamics of play: Including children with special needs in mainstreamed early childhood programs. *International Journal of Early Childhood*, 23, 50-57.

Singer, J.L., & Streiner, B.F. (1966). Imaginative content in the dreams and fantasy play of blind and sighted children. *Perceptual and Motor Skills*, 22, 475-482.

Strain, P. (1975). Increasing social play of severely retarded preschoolers with socio-dramatic activities. *Mental Retardation*, 13, 7-9.

Wortham, S.C., & Frost, J.L. (Eds.). (1990). *Playgrounds for young children: National survey and perspectives*. Reston, VA: AAHPERD.

Wilderness Adventure Trips

Glenn M. Roswal, Timothy P. Winter, Tom Collier, Eric Dresser,
Jill Hembree, Mark Singleton, James B. Wise

Wilderness adventure trips have been steadily gaining popularity in the United States as an exciting outdoor adventure activity. Wilderness trips combine active participation in an aesthetic outdoor context. Elements of risk enhance excitement and provide an avenue for stress relief. A carefully planned trip can contribute to increasing the self-esteem of participants while promoting healthy lifestyle choices. Additionally, the feeling of safety in numbers promotes an atmosphere both supportive and protective, particularly when participants are accompanied by friends and/or family.

Participants generally learn far more than simple outdoor skills. They learn the value of group communication and cooperation. They learn to work together toward a common goal and the value of helping one another. Outdoor recreation can make a unique contribution to the individual by providing opportunities to experience success while contributing to group functioning. Participants are able to learn to work together and together they learn to share feelings of group accomplishment.

Planning a trip for people with disabilities involves the same care and consideration as planning any outdoor adventure trip. Because of special medical or mobility needs, certain precautions should be considered. However, with a little extra care, effective and safe trips can be organized.

Materials presented in this article are composites of the principles and practices of three outstand-

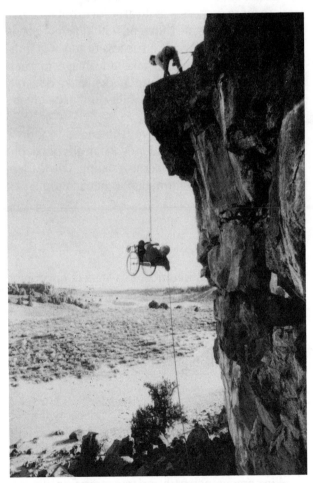

Wheelchair rappelling with the Idaho State C.W. HOG program makes an outdoor adventure trip truly exciting. *Photo credit: Brad Hicker, C.W. HOG.*

ing organizations providing wilderness adventure trips for people with disabilities:

Camp ASCCA (Alabama Special Camp for Children and Adults), P.O. Box 21 Jackson Gap, AL 36861

Cooperative Wilderness Handicapped Outdoor Group (C.W. HOG), Idaho State University, P.O. Box 8118, Pocatello, ID 83209

Nantahala Outdoor Center, 41 Highway 19 West, Bryson City, NC 28713

Organizing the Wilderness Adventure Trip

The purpose of any wilderness adventure trip should be to offer basic instruction and hands-on experience. The best way to meet this goal is through the careful planning of a series of small sequential successes. Success builds confidence, which in turn leads to more success. A critical point to remember is that all individuals are different, with different needs and different abilities. The successful trip will individualize the program to take advantage of each participant's abilities. Every individual has a different ability level, and adding a disability further heightens those differences.

Material presented here is intended to form a basic foundation for considering the needs of people with disabilities in the wilderness setting. Trip leaders should modify this information to fit each trip.

Liability

The first question most trip leaders encounter regards the liability implications of planning a trip for people with disabilities. The same principles that apply to planning trips for the general population apply to trips involving persons with disabilities. The key to avoiding liability problems is detailed preparation.

Trip leaders must develop the program by considering all possible situations. Accidents will most certainly happen, but contingencies developed will determine whether they result in inconveniences or disasters. There should be an adequate plan for handling emergency care and transportation, illness, injury, and fatigue. All participants and their families should be fully informed of all aspects of the trip,

including times, dates, telephone numbers, physical requirements, and risks. A good trip leader informs the group of trip details and anticipated plans of the trip beforehand, and makes each participant a vital part of the plan.

Trip leaders should make every reasonable effort to ensure safety of all participants on the trip. However, by definition, wilderness tripping is a risk activity. There are elements of danger that are beyond the control of the trip leader or professional outfitter in all outdoor adventure trips. To remove those risks would deprive participants of the excitement inherent in the activity.

Three practices used in the adventure recreation industry to defer liability are:

- Informed consent forms
- Common adventure trips
- Professional outfitters

A customary practice to transfer some liability to the group is the informed consent form. The form must be sufficiently detailed to inform participants of inherent dangers and risks associated with the trip. The consent form does not release the trip leader from liability, but does indicate that participants are aware of the hazards of the trip and agree to accept responsibility for their own actions. Participants in all activities should sign an informed consent form and participate in the trip at their own risk. For participants under 18 years of age and those unable to understand information contained in the form, the form should be cosigned by a parent or legal guardian.

An informed consent form and a release of liability form used by the Nantahala Outdoor Center are presented in Figures 1 and 2 in the appendix to this article. A program/activity consent form used by Camp ASCAA (Alabama Special Camp for Children and Adults) is presented in Figure 3 in the appendix.

Common adventure is a term which describes a situation where trip participants share in all aspects of the trip. Each member has specified responsibilities; each member is a part of the team effort to organize the trip. Group members participate in planning, preparation, decision-making, problem-solving, work details, risks, and liability associated with the trip. Although there are no designated or formal leaders, the trip is not leaderless. Usually more skilled participants emerge in natural leadership roles to help direct the group. Common adventure serves to minimize group costs and program liability while maximizing active participation by all trip participants. The minimum requirements of a common adventure include:

- Costs must be shared equally among all of the participants
- There are no paid guides or leaders.
- Skill level of participants must be relatively equal.
- Any instruction is provided gratuitously from one friend to another.
- All participants must have a shared responsibility for the success of the trip; no individual can be blamed for a bad trip.

Participants, regardless of the type of trip, must have an understanding of the activity, potential risks involved, and knowledge of required equipment. The information is shared among participants at a pretrip meeting at which much of the trip planning and decision making occurs and arrangements for transportation and activities are discussed. At the pretrip meeting, participants may decide to remove themselves from participation with the group.

A common adventure sign-up sheet may be used to make certain all group members are aware of their individual responsibilities and the responsibility of the group. Participants must be of legal age and capable of understanding, evaluating risks, and making decisions based on information available to them.

A common adventure sign-up sheet used by the Idaho State University Outdoor Program is presented in Figure 4 (see appendix). It is presented only as a sample and is not to be photocopied. Participants interested in using a common adventure sign-up sheet should consult a legal advisor for their particular area and program

A widespread practice in organizing many adventure wilderness trips is to utilize a professional outfitter. Selecting an outfitter defers many trip details and liability to the outfitter. However, trip leaders are still responsible for pretrip preparations and information sharing.

Selecting Outfitters

The most important aspect in planning a trip using a professional outfitter is selection of an appropriate outfitter. Considerations should include the reputation of the outfitter, safety record, years of experience in the field and with the particular site selected, quality of professional guides, and cost. Additionally, the outfitter should have past experience in successfully modifying trips to meet the needs of consumers with disabilities.

In particular, trip leaders should be able to satisfactorily answer the following questions concerning selection of the best outfitter.

- Is the professional outfitter a member of the appropriate professional organization, indicating it adheres to standard safety and training procedures?
- How many years has the outfitter been in business and does it retain its guide staff? An outfitter that cannot retain qualified guides indicates internal problems that may affect the quality of the trip.
- Is the cost consistent with other professional outfitters? Outfitters that set fees significantly lower than other outfitters may sound like a good deal, but often this indicates substandard guides or equipment.
- Are the guides knowledgeable and friendly? The quality of the guides will directly impact upon the experience of the group. Trip leaders should meet or speak with guide staff. Face-to-face contact can be a deciding factor in choosing the outfitter that is right for the group.
- Have other groups had a positive experience with the outfitter? The trip leader should consult with friends and colleagues on outfitters used for other groups.
- Is the equipment state-of-the-art? State-of-the-art equipment provides for safe, comfortable trips and reduced liability.
- Is the transportation safe and reliable? Many trips require transportation to access beginning and ending points. Trip leaders need to determine that the outfitter will be reliable in adhering to the predetermined schedule and that the members of the group will be comfortable and safe.
- What trip options does the outfitter provide? Some outfitters provide options from equipment only to a full package (guides, transportation, equipment, and meals) depending on needs of the group.

Trip leaders should remember that outfitters are there to serve the needs of consumers. The most direct method in selecting an outfitter is to talk with the outfitter and determine willingness and ability to accommodate the needs of the group.

Trip leaders may consult the resource list in this article to locate organizations with information regarding professional outfitters.

Campers at Camp ASCCA learn rapelling skills on the tower before graduating to trips on Cheaha Mountain. *Photo credit: Lisa McLaughlin, Camp ASCCA.*

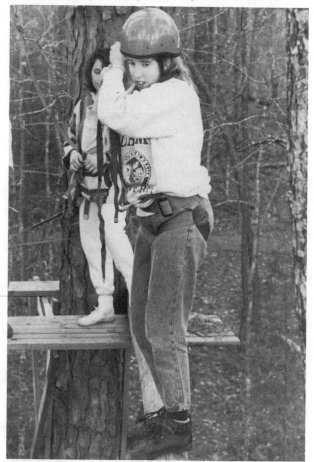

Safety and Risk Management

Risk management procedures should be used to make all outdoor activities as safe as possible. Risk management involves three steps:

- Identification of potential risks.
- Risk evaluation.
- Resolution.

The first step involves identification of likely risks in the activity (loss or damage of equipment, climber fatigue). Risk identification may entail consideration of the individual's disability, the activity environment (inclement weather), equipment malfunction, and instruction and supervision. Risk evaluation involves decision-making on the likelihood of a risk that could lead to injury. Risk resolution can include removing hazards, reducing risks, accepting risks, or transferring risks.

Risk management involves periodic inspection of equipment, continual evaluation of weather conditions, and frequent stops to minimize fatigue. Once guidelines are established, it is important for trip leaders to adhere to those guidelines. Wilderness adventure trips are not places for increasing risks through peer pressure and pumped up egos.

Medical Considerations

Wilderness adventure trips with consumers with disabilities involve special consideration of medical needs. It is advisable to have participants complete a medical form indicating activity restrictions, medications, allergies, etc. The medical information section of the Camp ASCCA application and a Camp ASCCA medical care waiver form are presented in Figures 5 and 6 (see appendix).

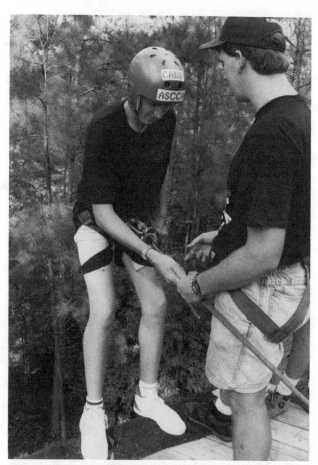

Low ropes courses (12-15 feet off the ground) are excellent activities to develop confidence for wilderness trips. *Photo credit: Holly Heath, CAMP ASCCA*

Funding the Trip

There are basically two ways to fund a wilderness adventure trip:

- Consumers pay for all the costs of the trip through fees.
- Trip leader raises external funds to sponsor the trip.

The most time-efficient method of conducting a trip is by passing all trip costs to consumers. Generally, consumers feel greater ownership in the trip and appreciate its value if they play a part in paying for the trip.

When consumers are unable to pay trip fees, the trip leader may turn to soliciting external funds to sponsor the trip. A few guidelines to consider are:

- All fund-raising activities should present persons with disabilities engaged in productive activities. Although raising funds through sympathy may be effective, it is counterproductive in spreading the message that persons with disabilities are capable of outdoor adventure recreational activity.
- Trip leaders should reinforce sponsors by returning something of value in return for a contribution. Follow-up reinforcement that makes the sponsor feel a part of the trip is an effective method of encouraging continued sponsorship.
- Fund raising should always be conducted in a professional manner depicting the disabled group and consumer in a positive image.

Some fund raising tips to consider are:

- Personal contacts should be developed; sometimes it is who you know that counts.
- Fund raisers should strive for one-on-one interaction with prospective donors.
- Slides and pictures of participants in action tend to gain and hold people's attention. Pictures of local participants increase the chance of personal recognition and interaction.
- Trip participants should be involved in promoting the program. A positive disabled consumer is a very effective salesperson.
- Trip leaders should be flexible and creative. Adapting to the needs of a sponsor increases the likelihood of funding.
- Donors and sponsors should be treated as valuable resources that are a vital part of the program.
- There should always be a follow-up (written or verbal) after trip completion.

Integration with Nondisabled Peers

The goal of an outdoor adventure recreation program for people with disabilities should be eventual integration of the disabled consumer into recreational activities with nondisabled peers. This is best accomplished when trip leaders carefully organize the program to take advantage of the capabilities of all participants.

The following suggestions are offered to facilitate the process.

- Participants and activities should be placed in a real world context, not contrived situations. Outdoor recreation is a powerful tool because the outdoors is uncompromising. People must learn how to work cooperatively in realistically appraising capabilities and limitations.
- Activities should be adapted only when necessary. Adaptations can inhibit integration with nondisabled peers.
- When modifications are necessary, equipment rather than activity should be adapted. The trip leader should attempt to preserve inherent risks that make the activity challenging.
- Disabled consumers should be asked to assume responsibility as a part of the group. Being a part of a group means each person is responsible for the success of the group in meeting established goals. When group members accept responsibility for their actions, they learn to take control of their lives.
- Whenever possible, friends and family should be involved, thereby enhancing potential for future trips. The nature of the wilderness trip necessitates assistance from and dependence on all group members.

Planning a Wilderness Trip

Planning, organizing, and implementing a wilderness trip for persons with disabilities is a tremendous opportunity often overlooked by the outdoor industry as well as by many in service delivery positions to the disabled community. Often there is a perception that wilderness trips are too strenuous or sites are inaccessible. Some trips can be both strenuous and full of accessibility problems, but with proper preparations a suitable trip can usually be found within a reasonable distance. Organizers should also consider that the most challenging programs may offer the greatest benefit. Often, gaining confidence in one's ability to be independent goes hand-in-hand with the benefits of exercise, the aesthetic natural and pristine beauty of the areas visited, and group cohesion.

Selecting the Group

Once the decision has been made to organize the trip, the next step is to examine the nature of the group. This may be predetermined through recruitment. One suggestion is to choose a group with like ability levels. This will tend to keep the group together rather than cause separation due to vast differences in walking speed or stamina. Trip leaders will need to determine the size of the group according to group needs, but should keep in mind that too many people can easily detract from the total group experience. A group of six or less participants might be a good number for the first time.

Site Selection

Choosing an appropriate site is the next task. Much of this will depend upon the nature of the

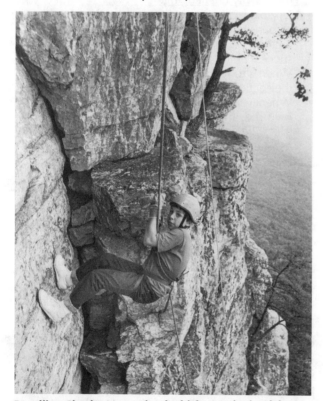

Rapelling Cheaha Mountain, the highest point in Alabama.
Photo credit: Glenn S. Phillips & John Friedenreich, Camp ASCCA

group. A trip serving persons with mobility impairments will require a nearly completely accessible trail. With a group of persons with developmental disabilities, the trip leader should look closely at the degree of difficulty of the trip, similar to organizing a trip with any first-time recreators.

- Is the trail full of steep climbs and switchbacks?
- Is it a relatively level lake trail?
- Have you done this activity before yourself?
- How long is the trail and what is the anticipated trip time?
- Are drop-off and pick-up points accessible?
- What is the availability of emergency medical services?

Checking available resources can answer many of these questions. Among those resources might be owners, managers of local outdoor stores, outdoor groups such as Sierra Clubs, program resource libraries, and rangers at the areas to be visited.

Trip leaders should visit and become familiar with all sites before the trip. Determinations as to accessibility, transportation access, level of skill difficulty, sun exposure, and distances to safe shelters must be considered.

A critical issue to answer on any outdoor adventure trip is the desire to balance accessibility with participation in a natural outdoor setting. The level of functional ability of participants with disabilities and the staffing assistance available will be determining factors in this decision.

Selecting a Date

The decision setting the time of the trip has an impact for several reasons.

- Does the trip involve cold weather camping? If so, the amount of gear and weight increases.
- Is the trip designed to catch peak fall colors?
- For waterfall trails, is the trip during a time water is flowing? Is water apt to be too high?
- Is the weather too cold or too hot for the type of group?

Clothing and Equipment

A great deal of information is available on selecting clothing and equipment. Trip leaders should do some research on types of equipment necessary for each particular trip. Local resources are a ready

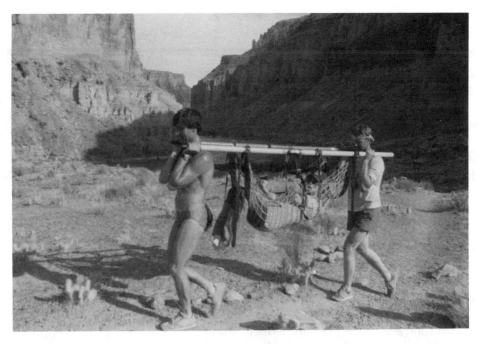

Hiking the Grand Canyon
with assistance.
Photo Credit:
Tom Whittaker, C.W. HOG.

source for this information. Trip leaders should decide what they will provide and what participants will provide. Experience indicates that few participants are able to provide much beyond their own personal clothing, and therefore, arrangements should be considered for providing everything from backpacks, tents, and stoves to sleeping bags, pads, and rain gear. Often equipment can be borrowed from stores, universities, camps, Boy Scouts, etc. A suggested clothing and equipment list for summer activities and a list for winter activities (prepared by C.W. HOG), are presented in Figures 7 and 8 (see appendix).

Staffing

Putting together a team of people that can be trusted will go a long way toward making the job of the trip leader easier. It is certainly an advantage to have staff who either know the participants or are familiar with their particular disability. Ratios of staff to persons with disabilities should be determined by factors such as the amount of assistance necessary and the functional level of the group. A fairly high functioning group may be fine at 3:1 or 4:1 participant to staff ratio, whereas a group of individuals with visual impairment may require a 1:1 ratio. Trip leaders need to examine all situations that may arise before making a decision.

It is important that staff include persons with technical expertise, for example, experienced backpackers, climbers, campers, etc. It is desirable that at least one person hold certification by a recognized

professional organization. Additionally, at least one staff person should hold current CPR, first aid, and emergency medical service certification.

In cases of more severely involved persons with disabilities, trip leaders should consider adding a nurse, therapist, or physician to the group. It is suggested that individuals with more severe disability, who require a care provider in their everyday life, consider bringing that care provider on the trip. This not only improves medical and self-help care but, if the care provider engages in the activity, it increases the likelihood of participation in future trips.

Program

Ideally, it would be best to meet the group once or twice prior to the trip. By allowing group input into the entire process, participants become a part of the trip and enjoy more of the fun and benefits. Their input into selection of site, equipment, date, etc. will help generate added enthusiasm. In many cases, the trip will be a first-time experience for many participants so a short two-day, one-night trip is recommended. This could be coordinated with a first night accessible campsite and camp-out prior to departing the next morning. This does not rush things, helps participants get acclimated to the outdoors, and allows plenty of time to organize equipment.

If trip leaders have not had opportunities to go over actual on-site trip arrangements, at least one to one and a half hours should be allowed for most groups to do this. Participants should be divided into teams of two to four people, with each team responsible for their tents, poles, food, etc. Equipment can be split up so weights are equal for all participants. In backpacking, packs should not weigh over 40 lbs. per person for a beginning backpacker.

Volunteers can be utilized by buddying them with specific individuals with disabilities. They should check to make sure everything is packed and help evaluate the amount of clothes and toiletries each camper is bringing.

When the trip begins, it is a good idea to have one staff lead the group and another stay in the rear. Trip leaders need to be aware of the need for scheduled stops for water and snacks, as well as to check the group for problems.

Upon arrival at the campsite, all participants (disabled and able-bodied) should assist in setting up tents and the cooking area, as well as gathering firewood. Have teams assigned specific duties to help promote group unity as well as to make sure the site is secure.

If the trip is designed to be longer than an overnight or weekend trip, it will require greater participation. Problems and solutions should be anticipated well in advance of the trip. Trip leaders should always be flexible and approach all problems with a positive attitude. See Figure 9 in the appendix for a sample planning checklist.

The program should involve a series of sequential small successes, that is, activities that meet small, easily obtainable challenges followed by increasingly more difficult challenges. A beginning level climbing and rappelling trip, for example, might include:

- Stage 1: Equipment knowledge and use
- Stage 2: Basic climbing and rappelling techniques at the ground level
- Stage 3: Experience on a 15-foot rappelling tower
- Stage 4: Experience on a 30-foot tower
- Stage 5: Mountain climbing trip

Small successes for individuals will make a wilderness adventure trip a big success for everyone!

Resource Organizations

These organizations provide wilderness adventure activities for persons with disabilities.

Alternate Mobility Adventure Seekers (AMAS), Boise State University, 1910 University Drive, Boise, Idaho 83725 (208) 385-3030

Bay Area Outreach and Recreation Program Inc. (BORP), 605 Eshleman Hall, Berkeley, CA 94720 (415) 849-4663

Breckenridge Outdoor Education Center (chapter of NHS), P.O. Box 697, Breckenridge, CO 80424 (303) 453-6422

Camp ASCCA, P.O. Box 21, Jackson Gap, AL

Challenge Alaska, Pat Reinhart, P.O. Box 110065, Anchorage, AK 99511-0065 (907) 563-2658

C.W. HOG (Cooperative Wilderness Handicapped Outdoor Group), Box 8118 Student Union, Idaho State University, Pocatello, ID 83209 (208) 236-3912

Durango/Purgatory Handicapped Sports Association, P.O. Box 1884, Durango, CO 81320

Environmental Traveling Companions (ETC), Fort Mason Center, Building C Room 360, San Francisco, CA 94123 (415) 474-7662

Nantahala Outdoor Center, 41 Highway 19 West, Bryson City, NC 28713 (704) 488-2175

National Handicapped Sports, 451 Hungerford Drive, Suite 100, Rockville, MD 20850 (301) 217-0960

National Sports Center for the Disabled, P.O. Box 36, Winter Park, CO 80482 (303) 726-5514

North American Riding for the Handicapped Association (NARHA), P.O. Box 33150, Denver, CO 80233 (303) 452-1212

Paraplegics on Independent Nature Trips (POINT), 4101 Cummings, Bedford, TX 76201 (817) 267-3029

Recreation Unlimited, Inc., 3131 Chinden Blvd., Boise, ID 83714 (208) 336-3293

Shake-A-Leg, P.O. Box 1002, Newport, RI 02840 (401) 849-8898

Skiforall Foundation, 4105 East Madison Suite 3, Seattle, WA 98112-3231 (206) 328-3732

SOAR (Shared Outdoor Adventure Recreation), P.O. Box 14583, Portland, OR 97214 (503) 238-1613

S'PLORE (Special Populations Learning Outdoor Recreation & Education), 699 East South Temple Suite 120, Salt Lake City, UT 84102 (801) 363-7130

Wilderness Inquiry II, 1313 Fifth Street SE Box 84, Minneapolis, MN 55414 (612) 379-3858

NANTAHALA OUTDOOR CENTER

Date:_____ File #:_____   **PLEASE COMPLETE AND RETURN TO NOC**

Land Activity: _____

Welcome to the NOC. In the interest of permitting the NOC to exist and to serve the outdoor community without fear of liability we ask you to join in this contract. The first part is for you to acknowledge that you understand and accept the risks involved in this outdoor activity and the second part is a release of liability. Your signature below indicates your understanding that the terms "outdoor activity" or "activity" encompass all aspects of the activity, including preliminary and subsequent matters such as, but not limited to, getting outfitted for the activity, maintaining, repairing, loading or unloading equipment or gear, and travel to and from the place of activity. IF, AFTER READING THIS DOCUMENT YOU CHOOSE NOT TO PARTICIPATE, WE WILL GIVE YOU A FULL REFUND.

ACKNOWLEDGMENT AND ASSUMPTION OF RISK — OUTDOOR ACTIVITIES

I understand and accept that outdoor activities such as hiking, backpacking, rock climbing, rappelling, bicycling or using a rope course expose me to numerous known and unanticipated risks which could result in personal injury, illness, death, or damage to myself or my property. Some of the risks or factors creating risk include, but are not limited to, the following:

— falling and breaking bones or sustaining some other severe injury;
— first aid or emergency treatment that may be rendered;
— accidents or illness in remote places without medical facilities;
— falling/fallen rocks;
— using ropes and other climbing equipment;
— hiking or walking in rugged terrain, including slippery rocks;
— injuries inflicted by animals, insects, reptiles or plants;
— hypothermia (cold) or hyperthermia (heat);
— the forces of nature including lightning, weather changes, river level changes and others not named;
— my physical condition, the physical exertion associated with outdoor activities;
— travel in a vehicle not driven by me.

I agree to accept and assume all responsibility for and risk of personal injury, illness, death or damage to myself or my property arising from my participation in this activity. My participation is voluntary; I choose to participate in spite of these named and other unnamed risks. I am solely responsible for deciding to engage in this activity and, while participating, for deciding whether to continue this activity.

I agree to obey all NOC rules and regulations while participating in this outdoor activity, and while on NOC property.

I have carefully read and I understand this Acknowledgment and Assumption of Risk. I also understand that I will be asked to read carefully, understand and sign a separate Release of Liability. I UNDERSTAND THAT IF, AFTER READING THIS DOCUMENT, I CHOOSE NOT TO PARTICIPATE, I WILL BE GIVEN A FULL REFUND.

_____   _____   _____
Participant's Signature   Printed Name   Date

_____   _____   _____
Parent or Guardian's Signature   Printed Name   Date
(if under 18 years of age)

Figure 1. Nantahala Outdoor Center informed consent form.

NANTAHALA OUTDOOR CENTER

RELEASE OF LIABILITY

I hereby acknowledge that I have read the Acknowledgment of Risk and have agreed to its terms. I fully understand that there are certain elements of danger inherent in recreational activities, and that participating in a recreational activity entails risk of loss of life, personal injury, and loss of or damage to property.

I understand and agree that the terms "recreational activity" and "activity" as used herein encompass all aspects of the activity, including preliminary and subsequent matters such as, but not limited to, getting outfitted for the activity, maintaining, repairing, loading and unloading boats, equipment or gear, and travel to and from the place of activity.

In consideration of Nantahala Outdoor Center, Inc. (NOC), furnishing services to enable me to participate in this activity, I hereby voluntarily release and forever discharge NOC and its officers, agents and employees from any and all liability or claims for any injury, illness, death, or damage to myself or my property arising out of or in any way connected with my participation in this activity. This release and discharge specifically includes, but is not limited to, liability or claims based upon the negligent acts or omissions of NOC or its officers, agents or employees.

I further agree, promise and covenant not to sue, assert or otherwise maintain any claim against NOC or its officers, agents or employees, for any injury, illness, death or damage to myself or my property arising from or in any way connected with my participation in this activity.

I further agree to indemnify and hold harmless the United States, The United States Forest Service, Tennessee Valley Authority, the State of Tennessee and their respective agents, servants and employees from any and all claims, demands, actions and judgements arising at any time out of or in any way connected with my use of the Nantahala, Chattooga, or Ocoee Rivers, or any government lands or rivers, and activities incidental thereto.

IN SIGNING THIS DOCUMENT, I FULLY RECOGNIZE THAT IF INJURY, ILLNESS, DEATH OR DAMAGE OCCURS TO ME WHILE I AM ENGAGED IN THIS ACTIVITY, I WILL HAVE NO RIGHT TO MAKE A CLAIM OR FILE A LAWSUIT AGAINST NOC OR ITS OFFICERS, AGENTS OR EMPLOYEES, EVEN IF THEY OR ANY OF THEM NEGLIGENTLY CAUSE MY INJURY, ILLNESS, DEATH OR DAMAGE.

I hereby grant NOC the right to use, for promotional purposes only, any photographs taken by them of me during my participation in their recreational activities.

I HAVE CAREFULLY READ THIS AGREEMENT AND FULLY UNDERSTAND ITS CONTENTS. I AM AWARE THAT THIS IS A RELEASE OF LIABILITY AND I SIGN IT OF MY OWN FREE WILL. I UNDERSTAND THAT IF, AFTER READING THIS DOCUMENT, I CHOOSE NOT TO PARTICIPATE IN THIS ACTIVITY, I WILL BE GIVEN A FULL REFUND.

_____   _____   _____
Participant's Signature   Printed Name   Date

_____   _____   _____
Parent or Guardian's Signature   Printed Name   Date
(if under 18 years of age)

Figure 2. Nantahala Outdoor Center release of liability form.

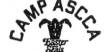

PROGRAM/ACTIVITY CONSENT

_____ _____
         (Camper Name)   (Session)

I hereby acknowledge that the above named camper is voluntarily participating in the camping, recreational and outdoor education activities at Camp ASCCA. I understand and acknowledge that she/he/I may be participating in the activities listed below:

PLEASE CHECK ACTIVITIES THAT INDIVIDUAL MAY **NOT** PARTICIPATE IN.

____Camping   ____Rock Climbing/Rappelling

____Arts & Crafts   ____Water Skiing

____Treehouse   ____Sailing

____Canoeing   ____Whitewater Canoe Trips

____Fishing   ____Swimming

____Horseback Riding   ____Ropes Course

____Riflery   ____Archery

____Photography   ____Nature Study/Demo Farms

____Hiking   ____Sports & Games

____Cooking   ____Pontoon Boat Riding

____Dancing   ____Gardening

____Field Trip Outside of Camp

I understand that he/she/I will be instructed in such areas prior to performance and will be supervised during such performance. I also recognize and fully understand that there are inherent dangers associated with the natural environment and risk involved through participation in such recreational activities that cannot be controlled.

In consideration of the Administrator and/or employees of Camp ASCCA enrolling my child/children/adult or me as a resident of said Camp, I do hereby release and forever discharge said Camp from any and all actions, causes or actions, claims and demands for upon, or by reason of any damage, loss or injury which heretofore have been made or which hereafter may be sustained by my child/children/adult or me in consequence of any accident occuring at said Camp.

I understand that this release/consent form will remain valid until otherwise revoked.

Signed: _____   Relationship:_____

Witness: _____   Date: _____

Figure 3. Camp ASCCA program/activity consent form.

IDAHO STATE UNIVERSITY OUTDOOR PROGRAM
COMMON ADVENTURE SIGN-UP SHEET

IMPORTANT NOTE: Before signing, read carefully the statements on front and back of this paper. Do not sign-up until you fully understand the statement and the risks of this trip. If you have any questions, please do not hesitate to ask.

Name of Trip_____Location_____

Departure Date_____Time_____Departure Place_____

Return Date _____

Pre-Trip Meeting: No _____ Yes _____ When _____ Where _____ Time _____

Pertinent Data:

Your signature below agrees to the following: I have read the statement on the reverse side of this document, and I acknowledge that I am acquainted with the dangers and risks of this trip. I, also, am of the appropriate skill level and physical condition to undertake the rigors of this trip. If I have any doubts of my physical or medical condition, I will seek medical advice. **I have made a careful decision that I am willing to accept and assume all risks.

Additionally, I have read the information on personal vehicles and understand that if I drive my own vehicle, I am responsible for my actions as well as providing proper insurance. I understand that ISU is not responsible for the safety of personal vehicles, nor does it provide insurance. I also understand that personal medical insurance is not provided, and I am responsible for obtaining proper insurance coverage.

I will not, nor will any of my heirs, hold the State of Idaho, Idaho State University, ISU Student Union Outdoor Program and their employees and volunteers and other participants liable for negligence or for any injuries or death or property loss. It is my specific intent and purpose to release, to idemnify, to hold harmless, and to forever discharge the State of Idaho, ISU, the ISU Student Union Outdoor Program, and their employees and volunteers, from all claims, demands, actions, or causes of action on account of my death or on account of any injury to me which may occur from my participation therein, as well as all activities incident thereto.

	Name (please sign)	Today's date	Phone	Can you bring your car?
1.				
2.				
3.				
4.				
5.				
6.				
7.				
8.				
9.				
10.				

Direct Questions to: _____ Phone _____

Before signing, carefully read reverse side

Figure 4. Idaho State University outdoor program common adventure sign-up sheet (not to be photocopied).

IMPORTANT INFORMATION ABOUT THIS TRIP—PLEASE READ BEFORE SIGNING

Common Adventurer: It is important that you understand that you are participating in this trip as a common adventurer. This means that you are aligning yourself with a group of people to share a common adventure or joint enterprise. The expenses of this trip are shared among all members. There are no paid guides. Any instruction or advice provided by any member of the group is given gratuitously in a spirit of cooperation. Members of the group do not hold one another or others liable for accidents.

On a common adventurer trip, everyone is expected to share in the responsibilities of the trip. The trip initiator (the person who posted the sign-up sheet) simply gets the idea for the trip off the ground. The rest of the group is expected to help plan, organize, cook, wash, load and unload vehicles, buy food, clean up equipment afterwards, etc. The success or failure of a common adventurer trip rests not in the hands of the trip initiator, or the ISU Outdoor Program, but rather in the hands of everyone that participates on the trip.

Any person is welcome to put up a common adventurer sign-up sheet and anyone who has sufficient experience required for the particular trip is welcome to sign up. The sign-up sheets on the trip bulletin board in the Outdoor Program work like a "ride board" that is commonly available on many college campuses. The "ride board" enables drivers and riders who are going to the same destination to get together. Drivers are able to find someone to share gas expenses and help with the driving and, at the same time, riders are able to find a way of reaching his/her desired destination. Common adventurer sign-up sheets, in turn, provide a means of getting people together to participate in an outdoor trip that might not have been possible if they had tried to do it alone. Idaho State University, then, simply provides a place for such trips to be initiated and has no responsibility for the safe conduct of the trip, nor does it officially sponsor such trips.

Risks: Please understand that when you participate in activities in the wild outdoors, you are risking your physical being. It is, however, impossible to list all of the dangers involved in this trip. The eventualities of injuries or death are so diverse that no one can second-guess everything that can go wrong. Before you go on the trip, you should become informed as much as possible about the inherent dangers and make sure that you are adequately prepared with the proper skills and equipment to minimize these dangers. Here are only some of the possibilities:

You can develop illness or die from: polluted water, spoiled food, improperly washed eating utensils; snake or other animal bites, and personal health complications such as strokes, appendicitis, etc.

You can also sustain injuries or die from: falling off cliffs; slipping and falling off wet or mossy boulders or trees; being caught in avalanches or flash floods; colliding with a vehicle, boat, rock, log, or tree; hit by lightning; hit by rocks falling in the mountains or canyons; attacked by bear, moose, or other wildlife; falling from faulty equipment such as fraid ropes; falling and receiving injuries from such climbing tools as ice axes, crampons, etc.; becoming entrapped in a kayak, raft, or canoe against a river boulder; entrapped in river hydraulics; falling through snow into underground streams; falling into streams or rivers and drowning; flipping boats in rapids, as well as many other possibilities.

The one important thing you should remember is that this trip is in an area far from medical attention. Help and evacuation can be days away. Often rescue, if possible, is difficult and expensive. If you must be rescued, you will be expected to bear the costs of the rescue.

Please do not go on this trip if you think it is perfectly safe. It is not. You and your fellow companions are expected to use common sense and make it safe for yourself and others. **Participate voluntarily and participate at your own risk.**

Responsibilities: In a common adventurer trip, you have very important responsibilities. These responsibilities include, among others: taking care of any personal medical concerns before trips and notifying other members of the group of potential medical or other problems, finding out the difficulty of the trip and realistically evaluating your abilities, learning about and obtaining proper clothing and equipment, obtaining proper insurance, finding out about risks and making careful decisions about participating in the trip and aspects of it, and helping in every way to make the trip safe for you and your companions.

Personal Vehicles and Insurance: If you drive or provide your own motor vehicle for transportation for the trip, you are responsible for your own acts and for the safety and security of your vehicle and those who ride with you. As a driver, you are **not** covered by insurance through Idaho State University. If you are a passenger in a group member's vehicle, Idaho State University is not responsible for the safety of such vehicle, nor does it provide any insurance coverage.

No personal medical insurance is provided. It is your responsibility to obtain proper personal medical and injury insurance.

Figure 4. Continued (not to be photocopied)

IV. MEDICAL INFORMATION

List all allergies (please include reaction and actions taken afterwards) _____

_____

Date of camper's last tetanus shot _____ Date last TB skin test _____ Results _____

Are camper's Immunizations up-to-date? yes _____ no _____

Has camper had any recent hospitalizations or illnesses? yes _____ no _____ If yes, please explain _____

_____

Can camper take aspirin or tylenol? _____

MEDICATIONS: Please list all medication**, dosages, and times medication is to be taken

Name of medication _____ Dosage _____ Times to be taken _____

_____   _____   _____

_____   _____   _____

_____   _____   _____

_____   _____   _____

_____   _____   _____

List any further medications on a separate sheet please.

PLEASE NOTE: Campers are expected to bring sufficient supplies of their medication, properly identified with complete directions for their use. Camp ASCCA will **not provide prescription medicines. Please send enough for the camper's entire stay plus several extras. Any extra medication will be returned.

Please list any problems (medical, behavioral or otherwise) of which we should be aware: _____

_____

_____

Figure 5. Camp ASCCA medical information section of camper application.

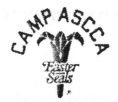

CAMP ASCCA
MEDICAL CARE AND PUBLICITY CONSENT
AND WAIVER FORM

CAMPER _____ SESSION _____

I hereby grant permission to the Camp Physician or his authorized representatives to furnish or arrange for the furnishing of such hospital and medical care as _____ might require during such time as he/she is a resident at Camp ASCCA. This
(Camper's name)
medical care shall include, but not be limited to, examinations, treatments, immunizations, injections, anesthesia, surgery, and other procedures, etc.

This permission is conditioned upon the understanding that in the event of serious illness, or accident, or in the event of a need for hospital services and/or major surgery, said person will use all reasonable efforts to contact the undersigned. Failure in such efforts, however, shall not prevent the provision of emergency treatment necessary for the best interest of the life and health of the said.

For and in consideration of said covenants, the camper and the undersigned hereby release, acquit and covenant to hold harmless the said Camp Physician and all other persons, firms, and corporations from all claims, damages, and causes of action of whatever nature which may accrue to the said camper or the undersigned, their heirs, executors, administrators and legal representatives and assigns, arising out of any of the above procedures.

Signed _____ Date _____ Witness _____
(Parent or Guardian)

Permission is also granted for said camper to be photographed, with such pictures and names to be used in public relations and fund raising efforts to promote programs of Camp ASCCA and the Alabama Easter Seal Society of the Alabama Society for Crippled Children and Adults, Inc.

Signed _____ Date _____ Witness _____
(Parent or Guardian)

Figure 6. Camp ASCCA medical care and publicity consent and waiver form.

SUGGESTED CLOTHING AND EQUIPMENT FOR SUMMER ACTIVITIES

Remember, on river trips all the things you bring must fit into one dry bag.

__ Wet Suit	__ Backpack
__ Extra Shoes or wet suit booties	__ Dry Bag
__ Wool socks	__ Life Jacket (Type III)
__ Rain gear (jacket & pants)	__ Sleeping bag
__ Shorts and/or swimsuit	__ Sleeping pad
__ Wool or pile pants & jacket	__ Tent
__ Gloves	__ Polypro underwear (top & bottom)
__ Stocking cap	__ Pillow
__ Comfortable dry clothes & shoes	__ Flashlight
__ Toothbrush	__ Eating utensils
__ Toothpaste	__ Knife
__ Hand lotion	__ Whistle
__ Contact Solution	__ Water Bottle
__ Towel & wash cloth	__ Insect repellent
__ Biodegradable soap & shampoo	__ Sunscreen
__ Razor	__ Chapstick
__ Brimmed hat	__ Sunglasses w/safety strap (rated 100% UV)
__ Windbreaker	__ Fishing gear & License
__ Medications	__ Camera

Remember, you may potentially be days from the nearest form of civilization. It is imperative that you have everything you need which may include medications, medical precautions and any special items necessary for a particular disability.

Figure 7. Cooperative Wilderness Handicapped Outdoor Group (C.W. HOG) suggested clothing and equipment for summer activities list.

SUGGESTED CLOTHING AND EQUIPMENT FOR WINTER ACTIVITIES

___ Balaclava (this is face mask/cap combination) or a wool hat and short muffler or scarf (for face or neck) - needs to cover ears.

___ Mittens or gloves -- preferably water resistant. (Sit skiers may wish to bring an extra pair to wear if the first pair gets wet.)

___ Footwear -- wool or polypropylene socks.
         -- Ski boots for stand-up skiers.
         -- Insulated over-the-ankle (preferably mid-calf) boots with non-slip sole for non-skiers and sit skiers, also suitable apres skiing activities.

___ Ski pants, wool pants or pile pants and sweater/jacket -- with wind resistant outer layer. (Cotton blue jeans are not recommended.)

___ Thermal underwear -- polypropylene top and bottom are recommended.

___ Turtleneck shirt and sweater or pullover -- wool, pile, fleece or polypropylene.

___ Socks (2 pairs) thin inner synthetic (nylon, orlon, etc.) socks worn under a pair of heavy wool socks.

___ Cotton handkerchief (works much better when wet than kleenex).

___ Chapstick, sunscreen lotion, regular lotion.

___ Goggles and/or sunglasses -- goggles are highly recommended for sit skiing.

___ Down parka/ski jacket - preferable water resistant.

___ Skis, boots, and poles for stand-up skiers.

___ * Backpack.

___ * Swim suit.

___ * Clothing for everyday when not skiing.

___ * Sleeping bag, pillow, sleeping pad.

___ * Bring an extra pair of socks and mittens to use for skiing when your others are drying out.

___ * Toiletries and medications.

___ * Water bottle, flashlight, bowl, silverware, cup.

___ * Camera and film.

It's often nice to slip into your sweats after skiing--or any clothing which is warm, loose and very comfortable after a hard day of skiing.

Dressing in "layers" is a good way to ski. You can remove or add layers as your body temperature changes.

* For overnight ski trips

Figure 8. Cooperative Wilderness Handicapped Outdoor Group (C.W. HOG) suggested clothing and quipment for winter activities list.

Sample Checklist for Planning a Wilderness Trip

Backpacking Trip

_____ Decide on objective of the trip
_____ Determine trip budget
_____ Determine approximate date, times, and location of trip
_____ Recruit and select group participants
_____ Recruit and select staff
_____ Schedule group meeting to decide location of trip, specific date and times, and individual participant responsibilities
_____ Decide on a backpack trail and accessible campsite
_____ Evaluate the trail prior to the trip for steepness, switchbacks, and water
_____ Make reservations if necessary
_____ Meet at least once with the group to determine
  • menu (keep it simple and nutritious)
  • equipment
  • transportation needs
  • assign partners and determine responsibilities
  • plan campfire games, songs, etc.
_____ Upon arrival at base campsite
  • put up tents first and secure campsite
  • collect firewood
  • prepare cook site
  • distribute equipment to each backpacker
  • explore area around campsite
_____ Discuss tomorrow's hike:
  • talk about the hike
  • how far you will go
  • what to do if there are problems; how to solve them
  • emergency procedures
_____ Pack backpacks (beginner packs should not weight over 40 pounds)
_____ On the day of the hike, everyone should check for proper shoes and socks and that backpacks loaded correctly; keep breakfast simple
_____ On the hike
  • start off with an easy pace (everyone will be excited)
  • hike about 5-7 miles the first day
  • hike less than 5 miles the next day (everyone will be sore)
  • have participants enjoy trip: the goal is not to survive, but to have fun
  • identify leaves, trees, birds, animals, plants, etc.
_____ Always bury waste and toilet paper; carry-out anything you brought in with you
_____ At the end of the trip collect all equipment; dry necessary pieces
_____ Schedule a wrap-up meeting to talk about the trip, share pictures and stories, and plan the next adventure

Figure 9. Sample checklist for planning a wilderness backpacking trip.